Effective Group Practice in Midwifery
Working with Women

Also of interest

Loss and Bereavement in Childbearing
Rosemary Mander
0–632–03826–8

The Law and the Midwife
Rosemary Jenkins
0–632–03629–X

Psychology of Pregnancy and Childbirth
Lorraine Sherr
0–632–03388–6

Effective Group Practice in Midwifery: Working with Women

Edited by
Lesley Page
MSc, RM, RN, RN (Canada), RNT, MT, BA
Professor of Midwifery Practice
Queen Charlotte's College of Health and Science
Thames Valley University, London
and
Centre for Midwifery Practice
Queen Charlotte's and Hammersmith Maternity Service
The Hammersmith Hospitals Trust
and
Thames Valley University, London

Part title illustrations by Heather Spears

**Blackwell
Science**

© 1995 by Lesley Page
Chapter 7 © 1994 Crown Copyright
Illustrations on Part title pages
© Heather Spears 1995

Blackwell Science Ltd
Editorial Offices:
Osney Mead, Oxford OX2 0EL
25 John Street, London WC1N 2BL
23 Ainslie Place, Edinburgh EH3 6AJ
238 Main Street, Cambridge,
   Massachusetts 02142, USA
54 University Street, Carlton,
   Victoria 3053, Australia

Other Editorial Offices:
Arnette Blackwell SA
1, rue de Lille, 75007 Paris
France

Blackwell Wissenschafts-Verlag GmbH
Kurfürstendamm 57
10707 Berlin, Germany

Blackwell MZV
Feldgasse 13, A-1238 Wien
Austria

First published 1995

Set by DP Photosetting, Aylesbury, Bucks
Printed and bound in Great Britain by
Hartnolis Ltd, Bodmin, Cornwall

DISTRIBUTORS

Marston Book Services Ltd
PO Box 87
Oxford OX2 0DT
(*Orders:* Tel: 01865 791155
          Fax: 01865 791927
          Telex: 837515)

USA
Blackwell Science, Inc.
238 Main Street
Cambridge, MA 02142
(*Orders:* Tel: 800 759-6102
          617 876-7000)

Canada
Times Mirror Professional Publishing, Ltd
130 Flaska Drive
Markham, Ontario L6G 1B8
(*Orders:* Tel: 800 268-4178
          416 470-6739)

Australia
Blackwell Science Pty Ltd
54 University Street
Carlton, Victoria 3053
(*Orders:* Tel: 03 347-5552)

A catalogue record for this book is available
from the British Library

ISBN 0–632–03825–X

Library of Congress
Cataloging in Publication Data
Effective group practice in midwifery: working
with women/edited by Lesley Page.
    Lesley Page.
       p. cm.
    Includes bibliographical references and
index.
    ISBN 0–632–03825–X
    1. Midwives—Practice. 2. Maternal
health services—Administration.
3. Maternal health care teams. 4. Patient
satisfaction. 5. Midwives—Practice—
Great Britain. 6. Maternal health services—
Great Britain—Administration. 7. Maternal
health care teams—Great Britain. I. Page,
Lesley
RG950.E36 1994
618.2'0233—dc20   94–26761
                                        CIP

Dedication

Dedicated to my family,
my husband Mark,
and my children Iain,
Anna and David,
and to the memory of my parents,
Ivy and Les,
with all my love.

Contents

List of Contributors and Advisers

Vicky Bailey, *RM, RGN*, Senior Midwife, Nottingham Health Authority, Nottingham.

Jean A. Ball, *DipN (Lond), MSc (Manc), RM, RGN*, Senior Teaching Fellow, Nuffield Institute for Health, University of Leeds, Leeds.

Rosslyn K. Bentley, *BA (Hons), Dip HSM, MHSM, Cert HEc*, Business Manager, Obstetrics and Gynaecology, Queen Charlotte's and Hammersmith Maternity Service, The Hammersmith Hospitals Trust, London.

Chris Bewley, *BEd (Hons), SRN, RM, ADM*, Midwife Teacher, North London College of Health Studies, London.

Agneta S. Bridges, *RGN, RM, BSc, MSc*, Clinical Midwifery Specialist, Maternity Unit, Farnborough Hospital, Bromley Hospitals NHS Trust.

Maggie Campbell, *BSc (Hons), RM, RGN*, Clinical Project Leader, The Centre for Midwifery Practice, Queen Charlotte's and Hammersmith Maternity Service, The Hammersmith Hospitals Trust, London.

Charles Chubb, *MB, BS, MRCGP*, General Practitioner, Kidlington Health Centre, Oxfordshire.

Pauline Cooke, *RGN/RSCN, RM, ADM, PGCEA*, Midwifery Lecturer/Practitioner with The Centre for Midwifery Practice, Queen Charlotte's and Hammersmith Maternity Service, The Hammersmith Hospitals Trust, and College of Health and Science, Thames Valley University, London.

Jackie Couves, *RGN, RM, ADM*, Midwife, Oxford.

M.G. Elder, *MB, ChB, MD, DSc, FRCS, FRCOG*, Professor of Obstetrics and Gynaecology, Hammersmith Hospital, London.

Caroline Flint, *SRN, SCM, ADM*, Honorary Professor, Thames Valley University, and Independent Midwife, London.

Maureen Freely, *AB Harvard magna cum laude 1974*, novelist and freelance journalist.

Jo Garcia, *BA, MSc*, Social Scientist, National Perinatal Epidemiology Unit, Radcliffe Infirmary, Oxford.

May Garvey, *RGN, RM, ADM, CHSM, DMS*, Head of Midwifery Services, Senior Nurse Manager, Supervisor of Midwives, Rochdale Healthcare NHS Trust, Greater Manchester.

Anne Jackson-Baker, *RGN, RM, ADM, Cert ED, MTD*, Director, Royal College of Midwives, English Board, Leeds.

Jenny Hewison, *MA (Cantab), MSc, PhD (Lond), CPsychol*, Senior Lecturer in Psychology, University of Leeds, Leeds.

Barbara Jones, *RGN, RM*, Directorate Nurse Manager for Obstetrics, Gynaecology and Midwifery, Hammersmith and Queen Charlotte's and Chelsea Hospitals, London.

Judith Lathlean, *BSc (Econ), MA, DPhil*, Professor of Education in Nursing and Director, General Nursing Council Trust Nurse Education Research Unit, Department of Educational Studies, University of Surrey.

Richard Lilford, *PhD, MRCOG, MRCP*, Professor of Obstetrics and Gynaecology, Chair, Institute of Epidemiology and Health Services Research, Leeds.

David Marlow, *AHSM*, Chief Executive, SHA Headquarters, London.

Helen Minns, *BA, RGN, RM, MTD*, Lecturer/Practioner, Department of Midwifery Education, John Radcliffe Maternity Unit, Oxford.

Mary Newburn, *BSc (Hons)*, Head of Policy Research, National Childbirth Trust, London.

Lesley Page, *MSc, RM, RN, RN (Canada), RNT, MT, BA*, Professor of Midwifery Practice, Queen Charlotte's College of Health and Science, Thames Valley University, London and The Centre for Midwifery Practice, Queen Charlotte's and Hammersmith Maternity Service, The Hammersmith Hospitals Trust, London.

James Piercey, *BSc, MSc*, Research Fellow, York Health Economics Consortium, York University.

Ian Seccombe, *BA, MA, PhD*, Senior Research Fellow, Institute of Manpower Studies, University of Sussex, Brighton.

Trudy Stevens, *SRN, SCM, BA (Cantab)*, Research Associate, The Centre for Midwifery Practice, Queen Charlotte's and Hammersmith Maternity Service, The Hammersmith Hospitals Trust, London.

John Stock, *BSc*, Research Fellow, Institute of Manpower Studies, University of Sussex, Brighton.

Ruth Wilkins, *BA, Solicitor, PhD*, Research Adviser, The Centre for Midwifery Practice, Queen Charlotte's and Hammersmith Maternity Service, The Hammersmith Hospitals Trust, London.

Foreword

In Britain, childbirth is experienced by 780 000 women a year – a large, important and sometimes vociferous constituency seeking change.

Aware of this, and the House of Commons Health Select Committee's report which showed that all was not well, I took the opportunity to break with Ministerial tradition to chair an expert group to bring about a radical change in the way maternity services are delivered to expectant mothers.

The group had to deal with very fundamental problems such as the place of women in society, the importance of women taking charge of their pregnancy and how services should be organized to meet their needs, ensuring the safe delivery of the child and the health of the mother. The group of experts augmented by the users of the service produced a report, *Changing Childbirth* which advocated radical reform. To achieve radical reform requires those who work in the NHS, one of the world's largest employers, to change their attitudes. Vested interests have to go. That is not easy to achieve, but now increasing numbers of midwives, obstetricians, paediatricians, anaesthetists, hospital trusts and purchasers are committed to change.

For those who still doubt the wisdom of change or who are unconvinced by the evidence, Professor Lesley Page, an academic, a true expert, a practising, practical midwife and an inspiring leader has edited this book which should both dispel doubts and convince the traditionalists that change is both inevitable and right for the mother and her child.

Now read on . . .

Baroness Cumberlege
Parliamentary Under Secretary
of State for Health

Preface

This book is intended for those who wish to develop organizational structures and cultures which allow us to provide sensitive and effective care and enable midwives to express their unique values, knowledge, skills and abilities in practice. Although written with midwives in mind, the book is aimed at all who are concerned with creating change in the maternity services, be they doctor, manager, executive, purchaser of maternity care or consumer.

For well over a decade now, policy documents from government, from professional organizations, and from consumer groups have highlighted the need for change in the maternity services. Likewise, research has indicated that there is a mismatch between what women want from maternity care and what the maternity services have been able or willing to provide. Government policy documents stated explicitly that there is a need both for continuity of care and to humanize the maternity services. Recently the Winterton Report (1992) and the Cumberlege Report (1993) have laid out in great detail a blueprint for the spirit and structure of the renewed maternity services. Women want more choice, continuity, and control in their care and the birth of their babies (Winterton Report, 1992). The maternity services should be woman centred, accessible, attractive and appropriate, as well as being effective and efficient (Cumberlege Report, 1993).

These two reports make it clear that fundamental reform is required in the maternity services. They have reviewed the purposes and values of maternity care, and set an agenda for change. This agenda requires that we transform the maternity services, and bring into practice such apparently simple things as kind, personal, sensitive and respectful care, and the possibility of the woman and her family getting to know and to trust the professionals who are caring for them. The development of practice which is focused on sensitivity to the individual and the skills of human caring will need to be based on a foundation of scientific understanding, evidence and evaluation of the effects of care.

This approach to practice will be required of all those who are caring for childbearing women and their families, but midwives especially will have a unique and important role to play. More will be expected of us than *ever*. Although midwives will become more independent in their practice, they will be required to work with other health professionals and health care workers within the maternity services in more productive and professional relationships. Independence of practice does not mean isolation. The new professional midwife will need to develop skills of referral and collaboration, and work as a peer to General Practitioners and Obstetricians in a unique but complementary way.

In calling for woman-centred maternity services, the Cumberlege Report (1993) requires that maternity care be flexible and responsive to the needs of individual families. This requirement will only be satisfied if the maternity service undergoes fundamental change. Individualized or personal care is a very difficult thing for institutions to provide, and may almost be seen as a contradiction in terms. But if midwifery is truly to mean working 'with women', it is axiomatic that it provide care which is responsive to individual needs. Working with women requires that we work in partnership with women, and know their hopes, dreams and fears, so that we may best look after their interests.

The transformative changes that are required will need clear thinking, real leadership, and commitment to commonly shared values. This book explores that need for transformative change and some approaches to creating and evaluating this change.

The book starts with the personal reflections of a woman who has had a number of experiences of pregnancy and birth. It shows the powerful effect of our care, powerful enough to do great harm as well as great good. The emotions of this chapter are naked: anger, confusion, fear, and great love and tenderness. It might seem like a sensational piece of journalism if it were not for the fact that many other women have spilled out these emotions and similar stories to the professionals, counsellors and researchers who have been willing to listen. Pregnancy and birth is a time of intense change, of psychological vulnerability, of learning to cherish and care for the newborn. Emotions can be intense, and reactions to insensitive care are often felt deeply, as are reactions to good and sensitive care.

This chapter is placed at the beginning of the book to emphasize the fact that our care is ultimately concerned with the personal and particular experience of individual women and their families. Our general systems, structures, and organizations are there for that individual and personal care. Maureen Freely's comment, at the end of her chapter, that with team midwifery care she felt strong and confident and full of joy with the love of her baby point to the real goal of our care. That goal is the support of this strength, confidence and joy of love at the beginning of the baby's life. The birth of a baby is also the birth of a mother, and usually of a father. It requires adaptation to new roles and responsibilities. Care should be sensitive to the need for this adaptation.

Other chapters draw on science, on the practical aspects of change and practice, and on reflection and description. It is this reflection and description which help us achieve a depth of understanding, and which will help us achieve both a scientific basis to our practice, and a reflective sensitivity to the needs of the families we care for, and our own needs in developing our practice.

This book is not only about finding a new structure for care, whether that be group practice, domino deliveries or team midwifery, it is also about seeking a new culture of care, a culture which values sensitivity, and caring human support.

Caring requires that we work in the best interests of those we serve. In other words, we should seek to do no harm, to understand the risks and benefits of the care we provide or offer, and to help those we care for make informed decisions about their own care. These decisions will include where to have the baby, who should provide care, and which tests and treatments are the best for the individuals concerned. So, not only skills, but also knowledge and understanding are part of our duty in caring. Thus, much of this book emphasizes the need for scholarship in midwifery, for reflection and for evaluation. Respectful, kind, considerate care requires personal skills, safe and effective care needs manual and diagnostic and scientific skills and knowledge. With both dimensions we can offer women and their families 'skilled companionship' (Campbell, 1984) on one of the most important and intense journeys of human life, the journey to loving, competent and healthy parenthood.

Likewise, *Effective Group Practice in Midwifery: Working with Women*, is intended as a guide to those who work within and lead the maternity services, in their journey to transforming organizations. Transforming organizations so that individual practitioners, both midwives and doctors might support healthy pregnancy and birth, while honouring the social, emotional and spiritual aspects. All those aspects which are so important to the baby, parents, family and to society in the birth and life of a new generation.

Lesley Page

Acknowledgements

My husband, Mark Starr, has encouraged, supported and helped: without him this book would not have been finished. Thanks also to Merle Mullings, who helped in bringing the manuscript together, and for the support of Lois Crooke, Head of the School of Health and Science, Thames Valley University. The ideas conveyed in this book are the result of work which has been supported by so many people it would be difficult to name them all. There are many travelling the same route. The work described needs many pioneers, each one of us as important and no more important than any other, for as in any pioneering work, we depend on each other.

I acknowledge the work of many midwives, doctors and others who are actively reforming the maternity services.

Lesley Page

Part 1
Background to Change

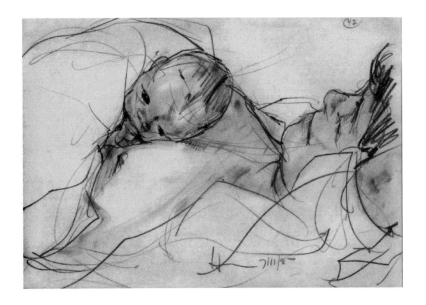

Chapter 1
Team Midwifery – A Personal Experience

Continuity of care. Care that is sensitive and flexible and woman-centred and performed in the right spirit. These are the aims of team midwifery. On paper, they look beautiful, irrefutable ... and vague. They tell you how team midwives should be – not how they put their fine new ideas into practice. They imply that the system in place produces care that is unco-ordinated, insensitive, inflexible, indifferent, author-itarian, and therefore undesirable, but they do not describe how this system can be modified to suit an individual's needs without ever endangering her or her baby.

What's it like to have the same team of midwives taking responsibility for you throughout pregnancy, during birth, and for the first ten days of your child's life? How is this type of care different from the standard treatment most women in this country can expect today? I offer my own story – not as a definitive answer to these questions, but as an illustra-tion. My experience may not be typical, but as anyone working in the field can tell you, neither is anyone else's. We might have a lot in common, but we are all special cases.

In 1991 I had the good fortune – some would say the luxury – of bringing a child into the world with the help of the Oxford City Team of Midwives. I got to know all six members of the team well in the course of my pregnancy, because they handled my routine antenatal visits on a rotating basis. They were on hand when I first booked into hospital, and during all my subsequent visits to the hospital clinic. They also supplied me with a number where I could reach the midwife on duty 24 hours a day. This meant that when I had a threatened miscarriage at 11 weeks, and some less serious (but potentially more dangerous) bleeding at 30 weeks, I was able to get the emergency treatment I needed simply by picking up the phone and ringing a woman whose voice I recognized and whose face I knew and whom I was fast coming to think of as a friend. There is no such thing as a faceless institution when you are in the care of team midwives.

My notes will tell you that my pregnancy passed without incident. The picture the team got was somewhat different. I was recently divorced, and living alone with my two children at the time. My main

3

source of income was a newspaper column; I was on a monthly retainer but had no contract and no right to maternity leave. I felt under pressure, therefore, to work right through the pregnancy and beyond. Frank, the father, was with me Friday through Sunday. He couldn't extend this time because he worked in another city. This led to a number of problems, not the least of them fatigue. Talking to the midwives about it all helped me come up with practical ideas for coping with my everyday difficulties. When I went in for my routine visits, one of the main things the midwives wanted to know was how I was pacing myself. I am not saying that I couldn't have managed without them. But I do know it was a comfort to have that kind of support. Also, I am sure that if things had begun to go wrong, they would have been able to pick up on it at once.

Three weeks before my due date, one of the midwives paid a home visit to explain the procedures of the birth to me and, also, because he was there, to Frank. She gave us general advice about early labour – when to get in touch with the team, how long to wait before going into hospital, what to take in when I went, and what I could look forward to in the way of pain relief. It was a two-way discussion. She didn't just give me the latest data on epidurals and pethidine and aromatherapy and what have you. She also wanted to know how I felt about these methods, what scare stories I had heard, and how they had influenced me. We discussed all of these before drafting a birth plan. Because it was a leisurely meeting, with the conversation meandering away from strictly medical matters in a way that it never seems to do in a surgery, the midwife had a pretty clear idea of the home emotional climate by the time she left. For example, although my notes would have told her that I had had my second child by caesarean section, she found out from me what kind of caesarean (an emergency operation performed in an atmosphere of farce and nearly ending in tragedy). She knew that I had decided to try for a vaginal delivery this time with some trepidation. On the one hand, I did not want to have another caesarean section unless it was medically necessary, because I remembered how long and draining the period of recovery had been. On the other, I did not want to harm the child in the way that my daughter had almost been harmed, so I was even more worried by the thought that a sympathetic midwife might postpone a necessary decision to operate out of a misguided desire to give me the kind of birth I wanted. I told the midwife that I wanted her and her colleagues to care for my baby, not my feelings. And of course, she took care of my feelings by assuring me that they would respect this wish.

My notes would have told her where Frank lived and what his profession was, but nothing else. When I was booking into the hospital, I did offer to give details about the obstetric history of the two children from his marriage. I thought this information could be as relevant as the information I gave about my own children, because they were, after all, as related to the child-to-be. I was told that the NHS had no interest in knowing. Because Frank was present at the home visit, he was able to pass on to the midwife information that was indeed relevant. Both of his previous children had been born three months premature by emergency caesarean. One had almost died. Because of these traumatic memories, he was apprehensive about attending the upcoming birth. Because of my own traumatic memories, I was even more worried at the prospect of going through a birth without him. The midwife's visit gave us the opportunity to discuss, in a reasonable and constructive manner, the possibility of his not attending. By the time the midwife left, we had agreed that he would attend. It's important to point out though, that she helped prepare herself by helping to prepare us. By the time she left, she knew that Frank meant well, and was going to do his best to help, but also that he was a nervous wreck and likely to turn into a basket case by the time we all met in the delivery room.

She also knew (and could have written a book!) about the many reasons why. Other sources of strain included (a) our children, who resented having been thrown together into a makeshift family (b) my job, rumoured to be under threat and (c) his ever-growing nervousness about having to leave me on my own to go to work.

Who knows? It may well be that I am a neurotic woman, but when I went to my next routine check-up, and told this same midwife that I was feeling worried about what would happen to me if I went into labour 'at the wrong time', I knew that she knew what I meant. In her eyes, if in no one else's, I was not *just* a neurotic woman.

It was a good ten days before my due date when I began to have contractions that were just a bit too painful to be dismissed by the name of Braxton Hicks. These continued intermittently, but never more frequently than every 20 minutes, until a good ten days after my due date. As nervous as I was about missing the signs and getting to hospital too late or alone, I was even more nervous about bothering the midwives with my every twinge of panic. They had enough to do anyway. I was afraid that if I overtaxed their kindness, I would alienate them, and so I made an effort to limit my calls. The midwives must have worked this out, because what happened is that *they* started ringing *me*.

By the time I was a week overdue, just about everyone at home was ready to get into one of those baskets. I asked the team for an induction. They were against it. They wanted me to wait a second week. But once again, the discussion was reasonable, and based on trust, as between friends. I saw their point of view, as I assume they appreciated my reasons. As a result, I did not become immersed in that Kafkaesque fury-paranoia that is so common amongst people who find their will pitted against that of a faceless institution. This meant that I gave due thought to the medical pros and cons of an induction. We weighed these against the wisdom of letting the home hysteria continue to rise unchecked. We settled for an induction ten days after the due date.

My contractions were coming fifteen minutes apart when I checked into hospital that Tuesday morning. Aileen, the midwife I knew best, was waiting for me in the delivery room. She explained that the induction would involve two stages (though as it turned out, labour established itself without my getting put on a drip). Once the procedure was clear to me, she called for a doctor to insert the gel to soften up my cervix. Even in my anxious and self-absorbed mood, I was able to note and marvel at the ease with which doctor and midwife co-operated. This was not what I had experienced in the past – but more on that later.

As labour slowly established itself, I sat in my chair next to the fetal monitor, chatting about this and that with Frank and Aileen. When the contractions came, the conversation stopped as Aileen talked me through the breathing. When they grew stronger (let's not hide behind euphemism: when they became close to unbearable) Frank held my shoulders and she held my hand. I remember thinking that they were my anchors. When, three hours on, I looked at Frank and said, 'Never again. Do you hear? Never, ever again!' Aileen said, 'Right. We're approaching the second stage. Onto the bed!'

I was only eight centimetres dilated but with a strong urge to push. I didn't have to try to convince Aileen, because I knew that she already knew I had run into this problem with my first child – and indeed had on that earlier occasion pushed too early, with the result that I had prolonged labour by another hour. I don't know if this is an illusion on my part, but at that point I felt that she knew exactly what was going on in my body and how it felt and what I must do in order to keep myself from making the same mistake again. In the end, though, it doesn't really matter if it was an illusion or not, because it was this conviction that made me listen to her very carefully and follow her every instruction to the letter.

The second stage took seven minutes – a blessing not just for Frank and me, but also for Aileen, as by this point Frank had given up on playing us soft, soothing music and had put on dissonant jazz, full blast. He could have been playing *The Sounds of Heavy Traffic* for all I cared. I had other things on my mind. The baby went straight onto my chest and is the only child whose eyes I saw and personality I got to know in advance of discovering the sex.

Helen was healthy and alert and took to the breast without hesitation. After the placenta had been delivered, I felt strong enough to have a shower, and then it was up to the ward, where I watched the other new mothers being subjected to the indifferent care of midwives on the shift, while I continued to get what looked like special treatment from the team midwives. In fact, if you added up the minutes of care we received, I probably took less time to care for, simply because my midwives knew who I was and what I had been through and so could use the shorthand of a working friendship.

The transition from hospital to home was an easy one because the midwife who saw to me in the ward was the same one who visited me the next day at home. It had been eight years since my last child. There were a number of basic babycare tasks, like topping and tailing, that I had forgotten. If the midwife had been a stranger, I might have been too embarrassed to ask her for help – or worried that if I admitted to a mothering flaw, she would dismiss me as a total incompetent. But because trust was so very established, I didn't think twice about it. I looked forward to the midwives' visits and was very sorry when they came to an end. Why? Because the care I received from them was care with a face and a memory and an ever-open ear. It made me feel like an active participant – and not, as I had been made to feel on other occasions, a vessel at the mercy of experts. It was not just woman-centred. It was man-centred. It was home- and family-centred even when we were in hospital. As far as I'm concerned, we got most of the benefits of a home birth without having to take any of the risks.

Of course there are many people who think of 'feelings' as existing beyond the scope of proper medical care. The job of the NHS is to look after our health. Hand-holding, ego-stroking, special pleading – these are expensive extras. To these sceptics I would say that team midwifery is not about providing expensive extras. It is a system based on the simple commonsensical idea that midwives can do a better job if their work is structured in such a way as to enable them to become acquainted with – and take responsibility for – their patients.

If you want to talk about expensive extras – accidents waiting to happen, like little problems that don't get nipped at the bud and so turn into big problems, and patients who are afraid to tell the truth, and midwives who routinely have to deal with crises without full information – then what you should really be examining is the system team midwifery seeks to replace: the system that most of us have come to think of as normal. If you want to understand the full value of continuous, co-ordinated, woman-centred care, all you have to do is spend some time in a 'normal' delivery ward.

I speak from embittered experience. When I say continuity of care is important, what I really mean is that I don't want anyone to have to go through what I went through when I had my first child at one of London's finest teaching hospitals. During the course of my pregnancy I never saw the same doctor twice. The admission procedure was brutal. First one woman 'prepped' me, then another gave me an enema, then, without forewarning, yet another broke my waters, gave me a shopping trolley, sent me into a vast Victorian chamber to give myself a shower, and forgot all about me. A midwife who just happened to be passing by eventually responded to my pulling of the emergency cord, and found me hanging onto the side of a claw-footed bathtub, groaning, and with labour fully established. She kindly put me into the care of a second stranger, who dispatched me to a labour room that was in charge of yet another new face. I didn't get to meet my midwife until I was approaching the second stage. She told me afterwards that she had shouted at me on purpose, to make me angry, because you needed to be really angry to push that baby out. I sort of liked her by this point – we had established a gruff kind of camaraderie – and given the circumstances, I almost saw her point. Certainly I had been too angry to care or even really notice when a group of students came rushing into the delivery room halfway through the birth. (I learned later that they were trying to avoid an inspection team from the board of midwives.)

We had a chance to get to know each other during the delivery of the placenta. I would have been happy to continue the conversation but, needless to say, she disappeared as soon as the doctor came to take care of the episiotomy. I did get to know the shift midwives on the ward during my week-long stay – although the relationships were not all happy. For example, the midwife on night duty didn't approve of breastfeeding, and secretly bottle fed all the breastfed babies in her care – this leading, of course, to ward-wide feeding problems. I took my own feeding problems home with me, and was not able to get much help in this or any other area from the district midwife who now took over. Her first action was to inspect my episiotomy, and decide that the stitches had to come out, then and there. Off to the kitchen, to sterilize a pair of scissors in a pot of boiling water. When I balked at the sight of her standing over me, flashing these scissors as she prepared to operate, she said, 'Open your legs, you stupid woman! You are a coward! Listen to what I am now telling you – I don't believe you are even woman enough to give birth!'

Well, actually, I had. And the baby was healthy, and so all, you might say, ended well. Except – birth is a beginning, remember? I don't think anyone could argue that this type of discontinuous care is the best way of propelling a woman into motherhood.

I don't think, either, that anyone in his right mind could argue that discontinuous, unco-ordinated care is medically safer. And again, I speak from experience. I gave birth to my second child in a hospital in Texas. The nurse on duty picked up fetal distress the moment she put me on the monitor, but because it was early Sunday morning, she didn't ring the doctor right away. She was more worried about overreacting, and giving the doctor a badly timed false alarm, than she was worried about the distressed baby. As it turned out, the doctor was furious when she finally got her call, because it was not a false alarm. (It turned out to be a marginal placenta praevia, with the beginning of the umbilical cord blocking the cervix.) She could not perform a caesarean herself, because she was only a family practitioner, so she had to call in a surgeon.

Because it was the first fine Sunday in May, most of the surgeons in the city were on the golf course. She finally located one who lived 30 miles out of the city centre. He, too, was furious when he finally got there. He wanted my doctor to tell him why she hadn't brought him in earlier. He sent me and about ten different drips and monitors into the lift, which then got stuck between two floors for what seemed like an eternity, but which was still not long enough for them to locate the anesthesiologist, who had mislaid his bleeper somewhere between the ninth and tenth holes at the local golf club (as he breathlessly explained to us when he made his eleventh hour appearance).

Count the number of expensive tragedies that very nearly happened that day simply because no one was sure who was responsible for what, simply because the system of care was not properly co-ordinated. The same applies to every system of obstetric care that is not woman-centred. The traditional methods may *look* right from the point of view of hospital administrators and their shift-workers, but to the woman herself, they feel about as safe as driving in someone else's blind spot. And yes, I'm afraid I can support my point with yet another story from my personal collection.

This one has to do with my fourth child's birth. I was no longer living in Oxford by now, and there were no midwife teams in operation in my new place of residence. I did see the same district midwife for half my routine checkups at my General Practitioner's surgery, but she had nothing to do with the team who took over my care when I went into hospital. Here a misunderstanding developed – partly because I had to go into the hospital in an ambulance after failing to awaken Frank. You will remember this is the man who has difficult pregnancies. When I had announced to him earlier that evening that I was experiencing con-tractions that were a bit too painful to be called Braxton Hicks, his first thought had been that we were looking forward to another twenty days of being on standby, like last time. And so he had foolishly decided to help his nerves with a tranquilliser. It's the sort of thing that is hard to explain to strangers in uniform when you're standing at the admissions desk and your contractions are coming two minutes apart.

This meant that they jumped to conclusions. They thought, right, it's Saturday night, which means the absent father probably couldn't wake up because he had a few too many. Let's find out if he's also abusive.

They checked my notes, on which someone (who? why? when? and for what reasons? no one knew) had written the words 'social problems'. I suggested that this could be because we had sought counselling after I found out I was pregnant, as the baby had been a surprise. 'Oh really?' said the nurse. 'Do you think your partner isn't here because the baby is unwanted?' It's not the sort of question you want to have to answer just after your waters have broken.

We had to go into pre-emergency mode at this point, because the water contained meconium. During the next two hours, while I watched the fetal monitor for signs of distress, three different people came to interrogate me about my home situation. Each one offered a visit from a social worker. All personal concern stopped, however, when they moved me into a delivery room, where the doctor and the midwife soon lost interest in my annoying groans and went into the corner for a long, desultory conversation about the pros and cons of holidays in Jersey.

I don't think I'll ever be able to hear the word Jersey again without feeling angry. I was very glad when, two hours before the birth, Frank finally turned up. From everyone else, though, it was a frosty and suspicious reception – even though he did as much as he had done the time before to help me keep going during the tricky, excruciating, but 'uneventful' birth. He was very angry to hear about the note in my notes, not to mention the ill-timed interrogation I had been subjected to. And so the war between the Faceless Institution and the Endangered Father began. When the innocent, unsuspecting district midwife made her first home visit the following day, he made a deliberate attempt to shock her by walking downstairs in his underwear saying, 'Hi. I'm the social problem.'

And it worked. She was shocked, and because she could see that I was shaking with anger, she assumed I was shaking with fear and so, naturally, was worried for my safety. She couldn't put Frank's piece of theatre into context, because she didn't know the context. She was meeting him for the first time at his worst. Now it was my turn to feel endangered. What would happen to me, to the baby, if the midwife decided I was not in control of my household? My first priority over the next week was not to keep things relaxed and quiet for me and the baby, but to make sure the house was looking perfect for the midwife's visit.

The irony is that this woman was just doing her job, and trying to do it well. If we had gotten to know each other under less fraught circumstances, we would have trusted each other. But once the misunderstanding started, it got large very fast. I suspected her of wanting to take the baby away; she suspected me of concealing social problems. It wasn't until the midwife's last visit that we had any sort of rapport, but it was too much too late by then to make up for lost trust. Of course I didn't need as much help as a first-time mother, but because I had had the benefit of team midwifery with my third child, this fourth (and last!) time I knew what I was missing. I've managed all right. I've kept the house going, and the six children, and I started work again before I even left hospital. But I know that the unco-ordinated, discontinuous, suspicious care added to my difficulties at a time when I needed all the help I could get.

What the team midwives did was the opposite. They gave me what I needed to get off to a running start. I may have been imagining things, but I always felt they were taking the long view – that their aim was not just to care for women during pregnancy and childbirth, and to watch over the baby's health during its first ten days, but to make sure that the mother had the confidence to meet the challenges that awaited her when she faced the world alone on Day Eleven. Life wasn't easy after the team midwives discharged me – I lost my newspaper column less than a week later. I had to go freelance. I had money problems, sleep problems, getting-dinner-on-the-table problems. I had to move the week before Christmas. But for once I was not having to use my inner resources to recover from a traumatic birth. I felt strong. I felt confident. I was overjoyed to have a new baby. For the first time in my life, I just got on with it.

Writing this chapter is my way of saying thanks.

Chapter 2
Putting Principles into Practice

Working with women

Midwife means 'with woman'. But what does this imply and how might we give meaning to the expression in modern day practice? The ideal in midwifery requires that we practise through a supportive relationship with the woman and her family, knowing them as individuals and knowing their particular needs, both personal and medical. Implicit in the term 'with woman' is the sense of being alongside and working in the best interests of the woman and her family.

Most present day systems of maternity care make these ideals difficult to achieve in practice, but there is a strong movement to renew the maternity services in a way which will enable midwives to again play a fuller part in maternity care. This movement is seen in many parts of the world, notably New Zealand, the United States and some provinces in Canada. It is particularly strong in Britain.

In Britain the Winterton Report (1992) set the scene for fundamental change. The Cumberlege Report (1993) then set an agenda which will require development and restructuring of midwifery practice within the maternity services in England. In the letter entitled 'women centred maternity services' and written by the Chief Nursing Officer for England, Yvonne Moores and the Director of Health Care within the NHS Management Executive, acceptance was made of the recommendations and a way forward to implement them was described (Executive letter 94(9)). A charter for women has been distributed informing them of their rights within the maternity services (DOH 1994a).

The Cumberlege Report focuses on the creation of woman-centred services flexible enough to respond to individual needs, and makes specific recommendations and sets targets for midwifery-led care. While the goal set out in the report is a general improvement in the maternity services, and the territorial attitude amongst the professions is deplored, the development of full midwifery practice is seen as an essential part of the renewed maternity services, and is something which many women want.

The report gives guidance on structures and patterns of practice which will enable midwives to practise fully and provide effective care. It is not prescriptive about models of practice, but it does provide specific organizational targets.

The idea that new structures are required to enable full midwifery practice is now generally accepted. Providing a new context for practice is regarded as one essential aspect of the process of change. I suggest the following criteria to guide the creation of new structures for midwifery practice:

- The midwife should be with the woman where and when wanted. To achieve this we must break down the barriers between hospital and community services, and move away from rigid shift systems.
- The majority of midwives should carry caseloads instead of staffing wards and departments. This requires that midwives take full responsibility for the midwifery care of a number of women being the lead professionals in a proportion of cases.

The structure of midwifery practice

I advocate group practice rather than team midwifery. The main difference between the two types of practice is that group practice involves a small number of midwives who carry a caseload, whereas team midwifery can involve much larger numbers of midwives and may be purely hospital based. Team midwifery has been implemented in such a meaningless way in some places that the term has become debased. Moreover group practice moves forward from the idea of team midwifery in that it implies the organization of a practice, rather than simply a shift of ward-based or community based staffing. This is a fundamental difference.

Personally I use group practice to mean the following:

- A group of midwives small enough to work in a cohesive and individually responsive way providing total midwifery care for a number of families in a community.
- Clinical leadership arising from a midwife or midwives working within the group, who are themselves engaged in clinical practice. In Britain this person may be a supervisor of midwives. (Supervisors of midwives are appointed by the regional health authorities in England and are responsible for the protection of the public. They are also expected to be guide, counsellor and friend of the midwife.)
- Each midwife within the group practice being the named midwife for a number of families. In other words, each midwife carries a caseload.
- The group practice midwives should manage their own time and their own resources.

The shift to a practice organization as the context of the midwife's daily work is a potent force for change. It is difficult to practise in this way without one's perspective being radically altered. When I practised in a small pilot project in Canada I was struck by the effects of this style of care not only on the families themselves, but also on me. First, there is a far greater sense of individual responsibility and accountability to individual women and their families. Second, the intensity of learning in this situation is dramatic. Last but not least, it was apparent that such simple things were particularly important to families: such things as being able to contact their midwife directly, or having enough time to talk in the clinic.

We cannot, however, just assume that because midwifery work has been restructured all will be well. Women do not only want the possibility of getting to know their midwife (or doctor), they also want care which is respectful, sensitive and kind (Cumberlege Report, 1993; p. 98), and they want competence in their care-givers. Group practices enable the development of a supportive relationship with the woman, and they allow the full use of midwifery skills, but they do not guarantee quality. Quality of care requires that the midwives practising in the group are able to provide sensitive and supportive care, and that their care is skilled and informed through knowledge and understanding. To understand how this sensitivity and skilled and knowledgable care is to be developed, it helps to understand the goals of our care. In this chapter I propose a goal of care, and have described the unique contribution midwives make to the achievement of that goal. Thinking about our care, and what we hope to achieve from it, requires that we challenge existing ideas about the outcomes expected of our care, and that we respond to what childbearing women and the public want from us, for we work in service to them. After describing the goal of care, I will propose three guiding principles of good practice.

The goal of our care

As midwives we aim to have parents leave us having felt cherished by our care, with pride in their accomplishment, and the joy of love in their hearts. Our goal is to ensure not only that a live and healthy mother and baby leave our care on discharge, but also that the mother, and wherever possible the baby's father, feel able to parent their baby competently and lovingly, with their physical and personal integrity intact. We should also keep in mind the long view of the parents' responsibility to their baby, their child, for many years to come. Our work is concerned with supporting parents in their adaptation to parenthood, as much as with providing physical care.

Technical skills, scientific knowledge, practical abilities, and good clinical judgement are all necessary for effective midwifery, but they are not in themselves sufficient. To be effective, knowledge and skill must be employed in the context of a relationship with the woman and her family. The midwife must be more than a clinician, she must also be a companion, a skilled companion (Campbell, 1984), to the woman on this journey to parenthood. If the woman and her partner are to accomplish the goals of this journey, they should begin parenting with high self esteem and self confidence.

Helping people become parents

With feelings of competence, and some sense of happiness and love for their baby, parents should be prepared for the demands of parenting, demands which they will need to meet for the rest of their lives. They will face sleepless nights, constant feeding and washing, complicated arrangements, lack of money, toddler tantrums, and then the natural challenges between teenage children and their parents as the child starts the process of separation. Good parenting will call for self denial, physical energy and emotional resilience, good and loving judgements, and an endless fount of love, tenderness, and faith in themselves as parents.

The ability to parent is affected by the parenting we have received, but also, I believe, by the experience of pregnancy and giving birth. The time around birth is a sensitive period of human life, of intense emotional growth and movement to different roles. The quality of professional care given at this time has powerful effects; effects that may be either constructive or destructive.

Midwives, and for that matter doctors too, must take into account this longer and broader view of birth. They must ensure that they are sensitive to the complex interplay of physical, social, emotional and spiritual needs of the woman and her family in pregnancy, birth and the early weeks of life.

Our view of birth is changing. We are gradually moving away from the perception of birth as a surgical event, and are increasingly becoming aware of the hazards of devaluing human support, of caring for women in faceless institutions, and of making birth too technical and sterile.

Renewing traditions

My introduction to midwifery began on a bitterly cold night. As a pupil midwife undertaking Part 2 of my midwifery training, I was on the district. I was off duty but had been asked to answer the telephone because the two midwives were out at separate home 'confinements'. The telephone rang at two in the morning. A woman I had met a few days earlier was in labour. I couldn't get hold of either of the trained midwives so I took a taxi to the house. It was in Edinburgh, and as the taxi dropped me off I was faced with a flight of about 40 steps. All the lights were on and the 'father-to-be' stood at the top of the stairs in his carpet slippers, anxious for my arrival. As I got to the top he greeted me, 'I'm glad you are here, the pains are coming every two minutes'. My heart skipped a beat, all my 'cases' had been in the hospital until now. At that I tripped up the last step, scattering the discreetly wrapped bedpan from my right hand, and my delivery bag from my left. Nonetheless, the anxious 'father-to-be' seemed to find my presence reassuring, and soon both a qualified midwife and a doctor appeared. What I remember next is the birth of the baby in a cosy bedroom in the soft light of the bedside lamp, the calm competent presence of skilled midwife and doctor, and, as soon as the baby was born, the other children spilling onto the bed, taking their sister into their arms, and marvelling at this everyday miracle of birth.

More home births followed, and left with me indelible memories. These memories were not of fear, but of calm and comfort, and of seeing women labour and give birth in the context of their everyday lives. I got to know these women as people, and I got to know their families too, in all their richness.

These memories have stayed with me, and have carried me through years of seeing birth at its worst: birth in sterile, angst-ridden delivery suites where the woman giving birth was a stranger, often alienated from those she loved, even her baby; pregnancy care in large over-crowded hospital clinics, with long waits and cursory examinations often by very junior doctors; precious days of early life with the newborn in overcrowded wards cared for by midwives or nurses stressed and fraught, with newborn families who became merely admissions and discharges. But memories from the past left blueprints, glimpses of possibilities for what it is we need to achieve now in our world which is altered so much from those earlier times.

In the chapters that follow there is much emphasis on traditional values. This is not to advocate a return to a golden age, for there were undoubtedly problems with our systems of care in the past. Times have changed, and so have the lives of women and professionals working in the maternity services. Nonetheless, we need to reinstate care that recognises enduring human needs, needs which seem to persist across cultures and across generations. These include the need to be supported in this most crucial transition of human life, to be accompanied by those who understand, to have companionship, words of praise and reas-surance and comforting touch at times like labour and birth, and to be cared for by a person you can trust to give you honest information, and to be competent in your care. This person should be the friend who works always with the best interests of you and your family at heart. We are not turning back the clock, but are finding new ways to meet these most enduring and fundamental of human needs, in ways which are appropriate to today's world and today's society.

These seem such simple needs, but they are not being met in our complex health care systems, where care is organized as though the childbearing woman is ill, and the care of obstetricians, highly trained specialists in surgery and complicated birth, is substituted for the skills of midwifery. The woman and her family pass through the hands of an assembly line of strangers, who, no matter how kind, competent, or caring, can never know her as a person, or follow through her care. In setting up new patterns of practice and renewing our midwifery skills I would suggest the following as guiding principles to practice.

Principles of practice

I propose three principles to guide midwifery practice:

(1) Choice, control and continuity.
(2) Effective care.
(3) Supporting the normal; detecting the abnormal.

Choice, control and continuity

In a lecture to midwives given in 1992 at the North London College of Health, Audrey Wise, member of parliament and member of the House of Commons Select Committee on the Health Services, commented on the fact that when women being cared for in the maternity services described particular wants, it was generally regarded as though they were being selfish, that all they actually needed was a live healthy baby, and anything above that was a luxury. I have certainly noted this phenomenon over many years both in Britain and in North America. And yet, as Audrey Wise commented, what sometimes appears as a want (wants are often considered to be something not entirely necessary) is often a deeply felt desire which is necessary to a woman, necessary to her health and personal integrity, and to her development as a mother.

As Oakley (1984) notes, many studies of women's experiences of the maternal and child health services carried out over the last 30 years show a considerable mismatch between what women want from the service and what the services are experienced as providing. This might seem paradoxical because birth is so much safer than it used to be; fewer babies and mothers are dying at birth than ever before. But it is not a paradox if we recognize women's wants as deeply felt needs. Women have been telling us that these deeply felt needs are not being met. In industrialized societies, where the holy grail has been absolute safety and the development of more and more technology, we have overlooked the meaning of birth in its social context. The social purpose of pregnancy and birth is preparation for becoming a mother (and vicariously for becoming a father), for taking on the responsibility of the care of another, highly vulnerable, person. The need for choice, control and continuity of carer should be viewed in that light.

The three Cs of choice, control and continuity are now an espoused principle of care in many organizations. But what do they mean? If we think about them carefully we know that giving them will mean profound changes in the personal professional care we provide and in the way our maternity services are organized. Recognizing the monumental change these needs call for might be why so many have gone to great lengths to argue that what women really want is not a midwife they know as friend, but is a shared philosophy, or good clear protocols, or good care plans.

Continuity

After reviewing the evidence, Chalmers, *et al.* (1989) concluded that systems that fail to provide continuity of care during pregnancy and childbirth should be abandoned. Fragmented care has certainly been highlighted as a problem for many years (Oakley, 1984). A face-to-face interview study carried out by MORI's Health Research Unit on behalf of the Expert Maternity Group found that continuity of care was regarded as very important by the women interviewed (Rudat, *et al.*, 1993).

Some, however, have argued that continuity is not a woman's highest priority, that above this she needs respectful, kind care, or to know her baby is healthy. Often this information has been gleaned from poorly conceived questionnaires which ask women to make choices between respect, kindness and communication, and continuity, forcing an artificial dichotomy. It is like asking somebody about to take a long trip whether they would rather take water or food!

So what do we mean when we say women want continuity? Women who know their midwife say things like 'we just felt very confident when you arrived', or 'things were really difficult until Jacky arrived but I knew she would help me', or 'I want someone I know and trust with me in labour'. Like the many women we met as an expert maternity group gathering information for the Cumberlege Report (1993), they talk about the reassurance they gained from seeing the 'familiar face' of their midwife or doctor. These are simple, understandable human needs, the needs and wants of people going through one of the most profound and intense events of human life. Seeing this need in this simple way helps us when we plan for the changes we are about to make in our organizations. It helps us avoid the trap of thinking that dividing midwives into ward based teams of 20, 30 or 40 will let us off the hook. If we really want to support women, this kind of change really will not help at all.

We provide continuity to give women real choice and control. We provide continuity so that there is someone, either midwife or doctor, who works with the woman and her family, one to one, getting to know her needs, giving information in a way that she understands and supporting her in making up her own mind. The choices to be made might be about her treatment, where she wants her baby, or who she wants as her lead clinician. We provide continuity to make sure there is someone the woman knows, who can be with her and comfort her and encourage her at times of need: someone to comfort her when she feels she cannot go on with her daily life as the fatigue and nausea of pregnancy seem too much to bear, when she feels at 40 weeks the baby will never come, when at six centimetres dilated she feels she has to have an epidural and wants to curse the world, and when, after nights of sleep deprivation she feels she will never make a mother, never have a normal life again.

The effect of continuity of care

Continuity of care is an important form of social support, and it seems that it is certainly likely to meet the perceived needs of women and to enhance their experience of care. But what of the effects of continuity on physical and psycho-social outcomes? Unfortunately, few team midwifery developments were evaluated and reported. The most important evaluation remains *The Know Your Midwife* project evaluation (Flint & Poulengeris, 1987). An early evaluation of the first women to be cared for by team midwives in the Kidlington Team in Oxford, conducted before woman had been booked right through the system, showed greater satisfaction with the pregnancy and birth of the baby where team care was given, and a statistically significant reduction in the use of analgesia and anaesthesia (Watson, 1990).

Continuity is important through all parts of pregnancy, birth and the postnatal period, but it is particularly critical during labour and birth itself. Think of the nature of labour and birth: there is nothing in human life to compare with it. Labour and giving birth require great physical and emotional endurance, they entail what is often excruciating pain. This is a time of taking on the responsibilities of mothering. Life will truly never be the same again. It is surprising that in the western world we continue to leave women unattended in labour, and when they are attended it is often by strangers, sometimes a large number of strangers. Continuity is not guaranteed even for the time of labour and birth itself.

One of the aims of group practices is to ensure that each woman has the one-to-one attention of a midwife for labour and birth. Overviews (or meta-analyses) of randomized clinical trials, indicate a strong effect of support in labour. The support in these trials was defined as providing continuous presence of a trained care-giver (midwife, nurse or doula), comforting touch, and words of reassurance.

Figure 2.1 shows the results of ten trials of moderate to high methodological quality from different parts of the world. Hodnett (1993a)

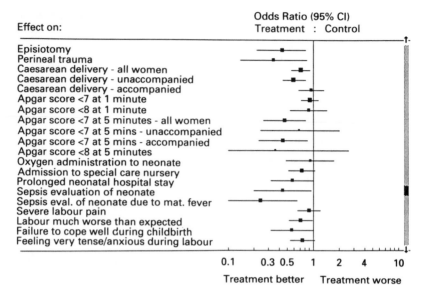

Fig. 2.1 Support from care-givers childbirth (10 trials reviewed). (Source: *Cochrane Collaboration Pregnancy and Childbirth Database.* Reproduced with permission of Update Software, Oxford.)

remarks that despite the disparate conditions under which the trials were conducted there was a remarkable similarity between the interventions as they were described. Each horizontal line represents the results of one trial (the shorter the line the more certain the result), and the oblong represents their combined results. The vertical line indicates the position around which the horizontal lines would cluster if the two treatments compared in the trials had similar effects; if a horizontal line touches the vertical line, it means that that particular trial found no clear difference between the two treatments. The position of the oblong to the left of the vertical line indicates that the treatment studied is beneficial (Cochrane Collaboration Pregnancy and Childbirth Database, 1993).

Thus if you look at Fig. 2.3 you will see that the provision of support during labour has a positive effect on problems during labour, on prolonged first stage of labour, on transfer between labour and delivery room and on operative vaginal delivery. This intervention also has, as Fig. 2.2 indicates, an effect on Apgar score of less than seven at five minutes, failure in midwife father relationship, on finding mothering difficult, and on non exclusive breastfeeding at six weeks postpartum. Figure 2.3 also shows a positive effect on the use of analgesia and anaesthesia in labour.

The evidence that human support can have an effect on physical as well as psycho-social outcomes indicates the need to have organizations

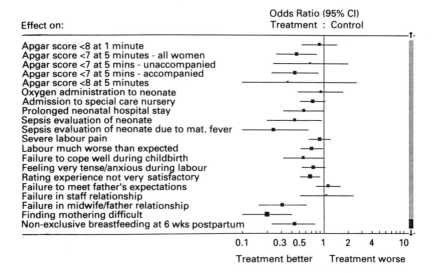

Fig. 2.2   Support from care-givers during childbirth (10 trials reviewed).
(Source: *Cochrane Collaboration Pregnancy and Childbirth Database.*
Reproduced with permission of Update Software, Oxford.)

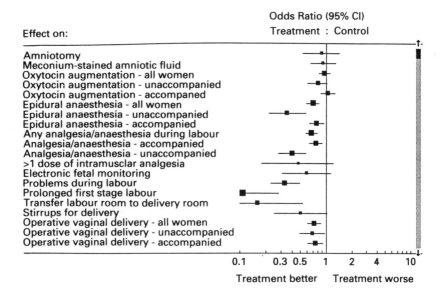

Fig. 2.3   Support from care-givers during childbirth (10 trials reviewed).
(Source: *Cochrane Collaboration Pregnancy and Childbirth Database.*
Reproduced with permission of Update Software, Oxford.)

where this support is possible, and where the principles of care should encompass this need. In many ways, this takes us back to the simple things, of staying with the woman in labour, of using words of praise and encouragement, of creating calm, of back rubbing and brow stroking and hand holding, of understanding that sitting and listening might be more important than the physical exam. These might be the most important things we can do for a woman. The evidence should certainly have us question very seriously the technical environment which exists in many hospitals, especially when that technical approach is not countered by adequate staffing and appropriate attitudes.

Control and choice

Control and choice are closely related to the question of satisfaction in childbirth, and although we often try to separate these concepts, they are so intertwined, and the psychological constructs are so complex, that it may be counterproductive to do so. Two important studies give some ideas of what 'control' and 'choice' mean to women. The first was a prospective study of 825 women (Green, et al., 1990). It was found in this study that contrary to common stereotypes, less-educated women did not want to hand over all control to the staff, and women of all educational levels were equally likely to subscribe to the ideal of avoiding drugs during labour. Furthermore, women who had high expectations were not bound to defeat and failure, as some have suggested. Instead, it was women who had low expectations who were more likely to have poor psychological outcomes.

The study was designed to assess the relationship between pre-ferences, expectations and experiences, and women's subsequent feelings. It used a variety of assessments of women's feelings after birth, including fulfilment, satisfaction with birth, emotional well-being and description of baby. The themes of information and control kept recurring throughout the results. Information seems to have been important at every stage. Women who did not feel in control were less likely to feel satisfied or fulfilled, and had low postnatal well-being scores (Green, et al., 1990).

Of particular importance for the purpose of our discussion here was the finding that decision-making was only one aspect of the perception of being in control. The results suggested that feeling in control related much more broadly to the sort of relationship that women felt they had with the staff. The authors concluded that although some obstetrical outcomes might inevitably result in a loss of control, the data indicated that minor interventions and particular psycho-social factors are also likely to lead to a feeling of a loss of control. The psycho-social factors included lack of information, lack of continuity of care and unsupportive staff.

A small but important retrospective study agrees with the findings of

Green, *et al.* (1990). This study, by Simkin (1991), explored the long-term impact of the birth experience on a group of twenty women 15–20 years after the birth of their first baby. These women reported memories that were still deeply felt and vivid. Those that were more satisfied thought that they had accomplished something very important, that they were in control, and that the birth experience contributed to their self confidence and self esteem. Also, they had positive associations with their doctors' and nurses' words and actions in labour. This link between a sense of control and later emotional well-being is an important one. Both studies tell us that the relationship with staff is an important factor affecting sense of control and memories of the birth experience.

Emotional well-being, absence of depression, and high self esteem are closely related. The work of Wolman, *et al.* (1993) casts light on these constructs. The authors conducted a randomized controlled study of 189 nulliparous women, with 92 randomized to the study group, to evaluate the effect of companionship from a doula (a trained lay support person) in labour and for the birth of the baby. The group receiving support – defined as companionship, comforting touch and words of praise and reassurance – attained higher self esteem scores and lower postpartum depression and anxiety ratings 6 weeks after delivery. The study took place in a community hospital in Johannesburg, South Africa, serving those unable to obtain private medical care. Only those who had no support person with them, as is common in that community, were invited to participate.

The Johannesburg setting may not be representative of other labour wards in other parts of the world. However, when taken with other evidence on the effect of support in childbirth, such as that contained in the *Cochrane Pregnancy and Childbirth Database* (Hodnett 1993a) we might safely conclude, as Wolman *et al.* have, that there is a need to attend to the psycho-social environment in which labour takes place in order to facilitate adaptation to parenthood.

Effective care

Am I doing the right thing here? Am I avoiding harm? What are the risks of this treatment or form of care? What are the pros and cons? How can I best convey the risks and benefits to this woman and her family? We've done it like this for ages, does it really work?

Our daily practice should be woven around with such questions, but in order to ask the right questions we need to know what it is we are trying to achieve. To ask the question 'Is my work effective?' we need to know the indicators that tell us we have succeeded. These indices will vary from place to place, time to time (Enkin, *et al.*, in press). If we are concerned with adaptation to parenthood as well as physical care, we shall be seeking to provide care which prevents depression, and increases self confidence, a sense of self integrity, and love for the baby.

In order to support physical integrity, we shall need to be concerned with maternal morbidity including feelings of ill health, or problems such as pain on intercourse, incontinence or backache. And of course, in our practice we seek to avoid morbidity to the baby, and death of baby or mother.

Having decided that in our care we wish to balance the outcomes of personal integrity, family integrity, adaptation to parenthood and physical well being, how do we then decide what works best? We should, of course, be constantly thinking about or reflecting on our own practice, noticing what seemed to work and what did not, looking at areas for improvement. This is extremely important, because it is the personal experience of particular women and families which is important, and we should seek to know the effect of our particular care, our personal communications, our style of work on those we care for and those we work with.

But we also need to inform our practice through science-based evidence, and through an accumulation of knowledge. This sounds so easy, but there are problems. Firstly, there is so much knowledge now, that it is difficult for any one practitioner to stay up-to-date. Secondly, how do we decide which evidence is good evidence, and thirdly, how do we avoid selecting evidence in a biased way so that it supports our point of view, and does not challenge deeply cherished beliefs?

We are aided in each of these areas by the evidence contained in *Effective Care in Pregnancy and Childbirth* (Chalmers, *et al.*, 1989) and the *Guide to Effective Care in Pregnancy and Childbirth* (Enkin, *et al.*, 1989). In addition, this work is available on computer disk, as the Cochrane Pregnancy and Childbirth Database (Enkin, *et al.*, 1993). The information contained in the disk is based on meta-analyses, or overviews, of studies and clinical trials from many parts of the world, from both published and unpublished work, which help us in understanding the effect of particular forms of care. The disk is regularly updated, and is easy to use. Much of the work in systematically reviewing the literature, in judging the quality of trials, and in pooling the effects of individual trials has been undertaken for us. The disk also provides recommendations for practice and for further research.

One complexity we face is in conveying the information to clients in an appropriate way. To help in this work the Midwives Information Resource Service (MIDIRS) is developing leaflets based in part on the Cochrane database. In addition, the MIDIRS Digest and MIDIRS database search, provide midwives with information about current research. Using information from this combination of sources, the Cochrane Collaboration and MIDIRS, is an extremely effective way of keeping up-to-date.

There are areas in which convincing evidence exists and practice still does not change. Clinicians (including midwives), either do not attempt or are unable to stay up-to-date, or else are reluctant to change. If the midwife is truly to be with the woman, acting in her best interests, she should know or seek out evidence, and inform those she cares for appropriately, and be willing to change her practice. One example here might be the use of the right suturing material and techniques. If, however, the clinical decision is outside the midwife's sphere of practice, if she is truly to be advocate for the woman, then she should make suggestions to the doctor and attempt to change the consensus view and influence clinical guidelines or protocols.

If we are truly committed to evidence-based practice, the implication is that we will go to great lengths to change in order to act on the best-available evidence. For example, it is difficult to see how we can ever justify leaving a woman alone in labour again when we are confronted with Hodnett's (1993c) review of the effect of trained support in labour.

However, even although we have a wealth of resources at our disposal, midwives still need to be able to interpret and evaluate the evidence for themselves, and to know at which point they should change practice, or challenge existing guidelines for practice. Because we have espoused a belief in using research in practice for some years now, it is very tempting to become very enthusiastic about the latest piece you have read in *The Daily Midwife* or wherever. Recently a colleague was told that she had probably caused a woman years of stress incontinence because she had allowed her to go on in the second stage of labour for just over two hours. We found the article on which this assertion was based and there was no mention of an association between length of second stage and incontinence, the variable described was difficult labour. We went to some lengths to explore the issue, finding no further information to help answer our question. Do we know whether or not length of second stage is associated with incontinence in later life? This provides a good example of the way we may read into findings those things we want to believe, and also of how it may be difficult to find evidence to give us all the answers to our clinical questions.

Critical appraisal of the evidence

'Critical appraisal is the process of appraising and interpreting evidence by systematically considering its validity, results and relevance to your own work' (CASP team, 1994).

Oxman *et al.* (1993) in their User's Guides recommend that the use of the medical literature is an essential tool for clinicians. Their guide to evidence-based medicine is applicable to midwifery. Evidence-based midwifery entails the same principles, that we start resolving clinical dilemmas by a careful definition of the problem, an efficient literature search, and a brief and efficient screening of articles. In their article they propose three questions:

'(1) Are the results of the study valid (true)?

(2) What are the results?

(3) Will the results help me in caring for my patients?'

(Oxman *et al.*, 1993, p. 2093):

They also suggest that resolving a clinical problem begins with a search for a valid overview or practice guideline. The paper I have quoted from gives a clear guide to using the medical literature. I recommend it to midwives who wish to develop their skills in this way.

But there is not always evidence available to guide our practice, so what do we do where no evidence exists, and perhaps where it will be impossible or at least impractical ever to find an answer? Do we change our practice anyway, perhaps on the basis of research where the evidence is inconclusive? Silverman (1994) comments on our preference to 'do something' in the face of uncertainty. This need to do something even when we have no evidence of benefit and no assessment of risk has characterized much of modern medicine.

Midwifery is characterized by 'watchful waiting' rather than 'do something to be on the safe side'. It is particularly important that we do not intervene unless there is evidence of benefit or unless the parents make a specific request. When appropriate, we should tell families of our uncertainty and let them make the decisions. Otherwise we should work on the premise of 'if in doubt leave it out'.

Supporting the normal; detecting the abnormal

The difference between midwifery and obstetrics has become hazy, particularly over recent decades. Although the two fields share a common goal, the work of each discipline is quite distinct. I am not advocating separatism; there can be no doubt that we need to work and collaborate closely. I am advocating that women with normal pregnancies should be cared for by midwives, and that, as has been recommended in the Cumberlege Report (1993), the midwife should be the lead clinician whenever possible where pregnancy is normal.

There are two reasons for this clear differentiation. First, it is uneconomical and inefficient to have such highly trained specialists (and sub-specialists) as obstetricians provide primary care. Secondly, midwives should possess the specialist skills, knowledge, and perspective, to care for women and their families where there are no problems, to promote health and normal processes, and to detect problems if they arise. Not only will this provide more effective care, but it should also bring the system of the maternity service, which is twisted towards an obstetrical model, back into balance.

The knowledge base of midwifery practice

If we are to practice effectively, and sensitively, and with an awareness of the potential impact of our practice on individual lives, families, and communities, we must take into account knowledge from a variety of disciplines.

The objective of interdisciplinary study is to develop theories of midwifery. These theories in turn help us in our clinical decision-making; help us to know how, in practice, we can best support women as they give birth to their babies.

Knowledge of the anthropological view of birth, for example, helps us gain an understanding of the meaning of birth, the part rituals play, and the effect of the dominant culture on the way pregnancy and birth are conducted and treated (Kitzinger, 1992). Similarly, some understanding of epidemiology (for example, that of cerebral palsy) is an essential backdrop to decision-making when we are looking after a woman and her unborn baby in labour. From psychology and sociology we gain some understanding of family formation, and the development of human relationships. The advanced practitioner of midwifery requires a matrix of knowledge and understanding which is the basis of midwifery theory.

Clinical judgement, diagnosis and decision making

Midwives will be challenged over the next few years to restore confidence in their abilities to use sound clinical judgement, to make diagnoses and clinical decisions, and to develop appropriate skills, in such a way that the woman herself is centrally involved and that physiological processes are supported wherever possible.

We use scientific knowledge and evidence of effectiveness to inform our practice, but eventually we all have to make clinical judgements, make decisions based on those judgements, and make decisions which take into account the values and wishes of particular families, and their medical history. Often these decisions fall into shades of grey rather than black and white.

Let me give an example of the complexity of decision-making in an everyday situation. Recently I was asked if I would look after a woman wanting a home delivery. I had been her midwife for the birth of her first baby and was keen to support her again. I particularly like looking after women when they have their babies at home. It always feels relaxed and is usually quite simple because you can concentrate on the relationship with the woman and her family, and do not need to think about communicating with a lot of other people, for example other doctors and midwives in the delivery suite. It just feels as though you can 'stick to the knitting' without interruption, and give relaxed and high quality support. I also like the endless cups of tea you can take before the woman's labour gets too intense! It is particularly nice when you have another midwife there for the birth, because a lot of camaraderie develops between you.

I have sorted out my own thoughts and knowledge of the comparative safety of birth at home versus hospital through looking at the work of Tew (1990) and Campbell & McFarlane (1987). Always ahead of time I make sure I am up-to-date on neonatal resuscitation, and other emergency measures.

So I was happy to be booked to undertake this home birth. But at some stage in the pregnancy, Laura (a fictitious name) spilled sugar in her urine, and her blood sugar was raised. So the question of the possibility of gestational diabetes was raised. This of course brought Laura, theoretically anyway, into a high risk category. Yet I knew that for this family, it was particularly important that Laura have her baby at home, and knew that going to hospital, for them, would be particularly stressful, and possibly even harmful. I sought all the evidence I could to try to work out the actual risks of 'gestational diabetes', and made a referral to the obstetrician. Laura herself had read all the literature, ahead of me, and through conversation I established that she had in depth knowledge of the 'disease', if it can be called that, of the reproducibility of tests, and so on. She also told me clearly that going to hospital would be a trauma to her, and she felt this would affect her labour and the health of the baby.

Although there was a theoretical possibility of shoulder dystocia, I was quite sure, from my abdominal palpation, that this baby was smaller than her first.

We decided to go ahead with the home birth and I let the local supervisor of midwives (see Chapter 1) know of our decision. All went well.

I cannot say, because all went well in this case that all women who might have gestational diabetes are safe to give birth at home. But for this situation, we had weighed up risks, the woman and her husband had made their own decision, and I had recognized their right to autonomy and their unique values. It would have been quite wrong to encourage this particular family to go to hospital to have their baby.

At the basis of these decisions was my knowledge of the apparent risks of home birth versus hospital birth, of the condition known as gestational diabetes and problems which might arise based on a review of the evidence, and medical advice, together with an examination of my own ethical stance and legal responsibilities in this situation. Then in the labour itself went my knowledge of assessment of progress of labour and maternal and fetal health, and the psychological and physical skills of support.

Differentiating the normal from the abnormal
It is the legal responsibility of the midwife in Britain to refer to a doctor if

there is a deviation from the normal. But what is normal? In reality the normal is usually defined by the culture within which we practise. In an organization with a strongly fearful or medical approach the normal may be defined very narrowly. There may be, for example, little tolerance for clinical judgement and allowing differing lengths of labour. In order to differentiate normal from abnormal we need to be able to predict the possibility of particular outcomes from research evidence. For example, what are the risks of pregnancy going beyond term? Or what are the associated outcomes with different lengths of labour? There are particular issues around commonly used interventions such as epidurals. Do we consider that the woman who is having an epidural anaesthetic is experiencing normal labour, and can her care still be directed by a midwife, or should her care be managed by medical staff? This is particularly important in maternity services where epidurals are frequent.

Much of the future work of practice development, scholarship and research in midwifery could usefully apply some challenge to current conventional definitions of normal.

Concern to preserve normal or physiological processes does not mean, however, that we should always allow nature to take its course. Although interventions should be used discriminatingly, there is a place for them.

Despite the inadequacy of risk assessment and prediction, part of the essential repertoire of midwifery skills is the ability to identify situations where more intensive surveillance is required, and situations where we should do everything possible to avoid any interference in the process of pregnancy and birth. We should also understand the difference between screening tests and diagnostic tests, the sensitivity and specificity of tests, and know the possibility of false positives or false negatives arising. This will help us understand which tests should be ordered and when, will help us counsel women when we gain consent, and will help in the interpretation of tests.

Avoiding particular screening procedures, such as continuous electronic fetal monitoring or ultrasound scans, will require that midwives regain or gain some clinical skills. For example, the effective use of intermittent auscultation (Page, 1993), or reliable abdominal palpation.

The skills of midwifery

Decision-making is in itself a central skill in differentiating between the normal and abnormal, in supporting normal processes wherever possible, and protecting the woman's sense of integrity. This requires an ability to integrate knowledge from evidence, from experience, and the use of clinical judgement. However, there are other skills associated with the support of normal processes in birth. Much of midwifery requires an ability for watchful waiting, while providing support for the woman. This support requires the abilities to be empathetic, to communicate effectively, to help the woman endure difficulties, but also to accept that for many women pregnancy and birth are a natural part of life, and that they need little advice, and are quite self-sufficient. Our skill is in deciding who needs particular support, and when and how it should be given. There is a balance between supporting a woman and making her dependent on the midwife.

In labour, which I highlight because it is a time of particular vulnerability, the skills of support require an ability to create calm, to use words and silence appropriately, and to use touch and massage sensitively and appropriately.

In labour our skill also lies in creating an environment where women might follow their instinct to move and find the most comfortable positions, and to relieve pain through support and presence and through other non-pharmacological methods. Often this is a matter of helping a woman contraction by contraction, and helping her remember that at the end she will see her baby.

The skills of communication are particularly important too, supporting the woman's personal autonomy particularly in labour, when there is a temptation to take over because the labouring woman is often in distress, and there is a tendency, as Kirkham (1989) found, to undertake what we think of as routine procedures, without even gaining the true consent of the woman, let alone involving her in the decision.

There is a paradox to be faced in respecting the woman's autonomy in labour, because labour induces an intense vulnerability in a woman, which is not surprising given the nature of the process. This vulnerability often has a woman almost change personality for a while and she may turn back on her enduring values and beliefs. For example, even although she has felt adamantly that she wished to avoid pharmacological pain relief or epidural there may be a moment when she changes her mind. This requires the ultimate in psychological sensitivity in the midwife, for the situation can go one of two ways. For some women it might be right to talk them out of using pain relief, for others the memory of the pain may become a real problem in the future.

Integration

Midwives integrate in their practice apparently simple things, like giving encouragement, support, comfort and companionship. But we also include more complex elements, such as interpreting the results of screening and diagnostic tests and an understanding of complex technology, for example fetal monitors. Midwives make complex decisions. It is in the balance of these skills of human support, in respecting the autonomy of the woman and helping her give birth in the way which is best for her, and these complex clinical skills that the art and science of midwifery lie. As midwives we work, as Davies & Evans (1991) reminds us, with heart, head and hands.

At the end of the day the acid test of effectiveness lies in the answers to these questions:

- Did I do all that I could to avoid harm?
- Did the family leave with good memories of their care?

Because there is one thing of which we can be sure: the woman, in particular, will carry those memories with her for the rest of her life, and the experience may cast a shadow over the parenting of the baby, at a crucial time. As a woman gives birth to her baby, she gives birth to herself as mother, and her partner becomes parent as well as lover. As midwives our care touches and affects these transformations, and we should be eternally sensitive to the possibility of good and harm in our effect on these individuals and their newly born families.

Chapter 3
Developing Scholarship in Practice

Introduction

In this chapter we explore the nature of scholarship and its meaning for midwifery. Examining the relationship between scientific theory and personal experience, we consider the professional development of midwives, searching for the hallmarks of excellence in midwifery practice, and offering strategies for the identification and perpetuation of good practice. Our strategies are drawn from personal experience and application in conventional and in innovative settings, and we use working examples to illustrate their use.

There is much talk about the theory/practice gap; we challenge the existence of such a gap and offer practical strategies which generate a theory/practice continuum. Within this continuum, theories are divined from practice, and, as practice changes, theories are overturned and replaced. Scholarship and practice are considered equal partners in the provision of excellent care, with one dependent on the other. But what is scholarship? What is excellent practice?

Scholarship and theory

Dictionary definitions of scholarship are unhelpful; they focus on the attainment of learning and, in the main, relate to children at school. Scholarship is also associated with higher learning; with the acquisition of debating and discussion skills and with the move into professionalism and higher education. It is also about acquiring new knowledge and reviewing existing knowledge. All of these things are important to midwives at the moment as we seek to raise the professional standing of midwifery, and as midwifery teaching moves into higher education. Even more important is the need to provide care for women and babies which is research-based and thoroughly evaluated.

So where does scholarship fit into this equation? Some would say that scholarly is the same as academic, but what is academic? Again, the dictionary definition is unhelpful; one meaning suggests that academic is 'cold, abstract, impractical, theoretical', all words which somehow fail to capture the ethos of midwifery. Definition of scholarship and academia may be problematic, but it is the business of neither to mystify nor obscure knowledge. Sadly, for many writers the hallmark of academia and scholarship lies in the use of incomprehensible language and jargon which bear little relationship to practice.

In both nursing and midwifery, there is a preoccupation with the 'theory/practice' gap. Some think that connections with academia and scholarship will take us away from the world of practice which we inhabit and in which we provide care. Perhaps we should consider what theory is and whether it has a part to play in developing scholarship in practice.

Theory has a number of purposes which move between the past, present and future. One purpose is to explain what is happening; to analyse and formulate a plan of action, a way of doing things, or an experience, with the aim of putting into words the actions and experiences in a form which can be readily understood. It is a way of giving meaning and understanding to everyday events. It also has another function, which is to explain and give an idea of the reality to someone who has not yet had the experience. This is its purpose in education; to explain to students, in a coherent way, some of the things they will see before they actually see them. Similarly, after the event, considering situations away from the practice area offers an opportunity to review and analyse an experience and put it into words. This process could be called theorizing.

There is a constant complaint that theory is what goes on in the classroom or the college of health studies and that it bears little resemblance to the real world of practice. Is it not then time to acknowledge that there will always be a theory/practice gap; that there should be a theory/practice gap, because the theory is explaining practice? As far as teaching students is concerned, we can never know whether in the week that we teach them about breech presentation they will see a woman whose baby is presenting by the breech. We can only teach theory and hope that theory is founded on up-to-date research and practice.

The final purpose of theory may be the stumbling block. From past experience and actions, practitioners may be convinced that what they are doing could be improved. This belief may lead to the generation of theories which need to be tried out. These theories may or may not be useful. Theories founded in this way must be checked out in practice; it is not acceptable to 'come up with a theory' and impose it without its being properly checked.

To be valid and to serve its purpose, midwifery theory must be analysed and evaluated in practice. It may come out of experience, that is, be retrospective, or may be creatively imagined and researched, that is, be prospective. These thoughts provide the beginnings of scholarship.

Generating theory from practice

By generating theories from practice, we will gain knowledge about the way midwives function, and what it is about individual practice that needs to be captured so that it can be appreciated and taught to others. Street (1992) suggests that much of what is important in both nursing and midwifery is an essence which has never been written down. She differentiates between medical knowledge, which achieves credibility by virtue of being written down and made scientific, and nursing knowledge. Although she describes nursing knowledge, much of what she says applies to midwifery. Our knowledge is often learned at first hand, by observation, by modelling, by oral traditions and story telling. Street (1992) notes that attempts to write down such knowledge have been received with contempt by nurses schooled in older traditions. The nursing process and nursing models are cases in point. The slavish documentation these systems entail may well result in a situation where filling in the documents occupies more time than giving care. Nurses respond with apathy towards the documentation and continue with their own systems of giving care, which remain unrecorded in a theoretical sense. In midwifery, there have been attempts to introduce 'the midwifery process' and models for midwifery, but these have largely been rebuffed (Hughes & Goldstone, 1989). The lack of documentation about the care provided throughout the ages by women and orientated to women obtains even more in midwifery, where the woman's experience of childbirth is not deemed worthy of study. Thus it seems that there is a wealth of knowledge available about midwifery which is largely untapped and which needs to be analysed and written down in order to preserve what is popularly known as a body of knowledge.

The identification of a body of midwifery knowledge is also central to the development of midwifery as a profession. But what constitutes a profession? Or for that matter, what constitutes a professional? Downie (1990) analyses the characteristics of a professional and concludes that in addition to the skills or expertise peculiar to that occupation, the professional has a broad knowledge base providing the ability to see the profession from a wider perspective. This broad perspective enables professionals to see how their skills relate to wider issues. More importantly, the professional attitude is characterized by continual development of knowledge and expertise based on a value system of integrity, honesty and independence.

Thus the development of the individual midwife, and the development of the profession hinge on a particular way of looking at things; particular ways of thinking. Professionals need to think in ways which use imagination, creativity and intuition, as well as using logical and rational reasoning. Using imagination and intuition, midwives will discover the existence of problems for themselves, rather than working on problems identified by others. Knowledge and expertise in a particular field can be called on to provide insight and identify new perspectives.

Research is certainly one way of exploring midwifery knowledge; Schön (1991) discusses the nature of research and suggests that professionals are increasingly disillusioned with researchers who have little to offer the practitioner faced with making clinical decisions in indeterminate zones of practice and conditions of uncertainty. Some aspects of midwifery practice can be researched using both qualitative and quantitative methods, but there are others which cannot necessarily be researched. Perhaps midwives need to think in new and different ways in order to identify and develop good practice.

Thinking in different ways

Many different ways of thinking have been described: for example, lateral thinking, problem solving, creative thinking, critical thinking. These are names for complex thought processes which some possess already, which some can develop, and which some have had knocked out of them by a system which has traditionally valued rational thought and an unquestioning following of instructions.

Dewey (1933) observes that the combination of problem solving and creative thinking leads to reflection and critical analysis. This view is echoed by Schön (1991), whose work on reflective practice offers scope for bridging the gap between what he terms the academic high ground and the swampy lowlands of actual practice.

Developing thinking skills means freeing oneself from prejudices and uncritically assimilated ideologies (Mezirow, 1989), and it is here that problems for scholarship in midwifery may be identified. McPeck (1981) argues that the core ingredient for effective critical thinking must be foundational knowledge. He further suggests that critical thinking is not a generalized skill and therefore cannot be taught as a distinct subject. How then, can the foundational knowledge required for a midwife be acquired without the accumulation of uncritically assimilated ideologies? How can midwives exercise freedom of thought and obtain a wide cognitive perspective within the constraints of policies and procedural guidelines? Midwifery is a profession in which there can be many right answers to the same problem. In clinical practice critical thinkers will not necessarily arrive at the same conclusions in identical situations. Perhaps the development of new thinking will allow us to accept multiple realities instead of searching for the definitive reality.

The old style of midwifery training produced midwives who were skilful in practical hands-on care. Having a degree in midwifery brings a different attitude, thinking and approach. The old apprenticeship system comes in for much criticism, but in our search for scholarship, perhaps we should consider an apprenticeship of the mind.

The word 'mentor' has been adopted in nursing and midwifery, and its meaning entirely changed. Originally, a mentor was a member of one's profession, usually older, very experienced and often in a position to aid advancement. The relationship was not official and often developed as a result of the mentor being seen as a role model. The mentor exercised an influence which derived largely from her own personality and charisma. This concept of mentorship allows for communication of much more than information about a profession. Love of the subject and a sense of its intrinsic worth are assimilated by those in close proximity to a midwife whose attitude and approach reflect humanity, respect and interest as well as expert practice.

In more general terms, scholarship can be developed by the creation of an enquiring atmosphere in which discussion, reading and research are acknowledged as a legitimate part of the midwife's remit. The organization and analysis of abstract ideas and the formulation of theoretical frameworks are the scholastic outcomes of examination of practice. However, once these frameworks have been devised, the emancipatory nature of critical thinking will ensure that they can be updated or overturned with the acquisition of new knowledge or insights.

How then, can we develop scholarship in midwifery? Both authors have experienced methods of developing scholarship in practice, one within the Centre for Midwifery Practice and one in a general educational position, and offer some practical applications of the methods currently in vogue.

Peer learning community

One of the key elements of the Centre for Midwifery Practice is:

> 'To implement an academic environment which encourages personal and professional development utilising a system of peer review and support, providing direct and sensitive feedback to individual midwives through audit of practice.'
>
> (Cooke, *et al.*, 1993)

The academic environment which we seek to support within the Centre may also be described as a peer learning community, a concept which Heron (1974) uses. Heron describes the qualities of its members as firstly, those who are self-directing, and thus determined and committed to what are conceived of as worthwhile objectives, to acceptable means of achieving them and to appropriate standards of performance. Secondly, its members are self-monitoring, where performance is evaluated in the light of an individual's standards. Thirdly, there is the quality of self-correction, where an individual's performance, standards, means and objectives are modified in the light of reflection and experience.

Reflection

The term 'reflection' has become very popular. Reflective groups and reflective diaries feature in most course requirements. We are urged to reflect on action and in action. There are numerous books and articles which seek to define reflection and extol its virtues. However, there is a danger that over exposure will lead to reflection falling out of fashion, without ever having been used properly. In reality many midwives would say they reflect anyway and they do not need a formalized process for reflection. However, the formal process of writing fulfils a number of purposes. Imagine writing a letter of explanation to someone you know. You would take great pains to ensure that you are explaining things correctly and that you leave no room for misunderstanding. This is different from reflecting on the bus or train on the way home from work where no-one else witnesses the results of your thinking. It is also different from the anguished reflection and replaying of painful events which is the aftermath of a traumatic encounter. On the bus or train, or in your anguish, if you do not write down your actions, feelings, intuitions etc., you think and anguish without benefit. If you think these things through and write something down, you have built a foundation. You may hate it later, but you have recorded your feelings and actions at

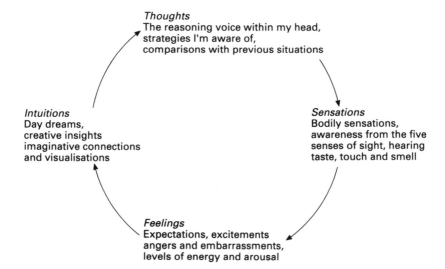

Fig. 3.1 A model for reflection (adapted from work by Barber, 1989).

The incident
I was a newly qualified staff midwife on a postnatal ward. I was working on a late shift with one other midwife who had qualified at the same time as I had. Towards the end of the shift, a newly delivered woman who sustained a primary postpartum haemorrhage was admitted from the delivery suite. She was conscious, with normal pulse, blood pressure and respirations. Her uterus was well-contracted and the amount of lochia was normal. She had a CVP line, and the readings were at the lower level of acceptable limits. A blood transfusion was in progress, and her drug chart showed that this was the third unit of four. The current transfusion was almost completed, and since the night staff would soon be taking over, my midwife colleague and I decided to send for the next unit of blood. This arrived and was put up. The woman's observations, including CVP were within normal limits. We handed over to the night staff.

The following morning, my colleague and I were called to the Supervisor of Midwives; the fourth unit of blood was only to have been used if the woman's condition had deteriorated, and we were called to account for our actions.

We had not seen the instructions concerning the fourth unit, which were written in a different part of the notes from the action and planning for the post delivery period. Furthermore, the CVP readings had been within, and on the lower side of normal limits. Our explanations were accepted and no further action was taken.

Thoughts
My actions had been based on what I thought were the instructions of the medical staff. The prescription sheet for the blood contained no proviso that the fourth unit should only be given if the woman's condition deteriorated. However, I have to be honest and say that I cannot have read the notes properly because I failed to see the specific instructions in the notes.

Feelings
I was horrified when the Supervisor sent for me. I could not imagine what I had done. I felt guilty and responsible when she pointed out what had happened, as I was very aware of the consequences of fluid overload following primary postpartum haemorrhage. I also felt that my knowledge

Fig. 3.2 Extract from a reflective diary.

the time. Figure 3.1 shows a model for reflection adapted from work by Barber (1989), and Fig. 3.2 gives an example of how a meaningful incident was recorded in a reflective diary.

Notice how the incident, which could have turned out disastrously, has been used to turn experience into learning. Here it appears in a reflective diary. It could also be brought up as a critical incident in a reflective group or any other group which seeks to review practice.

Another way of reflecting is by using critical incident analysis. This originated as part of aviation and piloting training, in which flying episodes were analyzed in order to perfect techniques. The strategy was base in the region of intensive care and fluid replacement, was lacking, although I knew from recent revision for my midwifery examinations that blood transfusion can continue until the CVP reading is normal. At the end of the incident, I felt inadequate and was made aware of the potential for making mistakes in midwifery.

Sensations
This is the part of reflection I find difficult. At the time, I remember, there were a number of babies crying but the general atmosphere of the ward was peaceful and calm. There was a faint smell of toast, made for one of the mothers who had missed supper. My hands smelt of freshly washed baby, as I had just bathed a baby.

Intuitions
As I went off duty, I had none of the sense of foreboding that often accompanies a situation in which one thinks there may be adverse consequences. In fact, on the contrary, both my colleague and I congratulated ourselves on our forward thinking in getting the blood before the night staff arrived. My conclusion is that I was not showing any intuition in this instance.

Thoughts
From this experience, I realize that I need to read notes more carefully. I made assumptions from what was written on the prescription sheet, and these were incorrect.

   Perhaps the notes need to be rethought so that instructions can be seen clearly and there is no room for confusion. Perhaps I should also strive for a more collaborative relationship with the delivery suite and medical staff in planning and implementing care, so that there is a two-way process, and good flow of information. Maybe, also, I should not assume that because there is another midwife on duty with me, we are bound to get everything right.

   I have learned not to make assumptions, and not to rely on two heads being better than one. I have also learned (or re-learned) the necessity for good interprofessional communication.

Fig. 3.2 (cont.)

used by Benner (1984) to observe and categorize nursing interventions and the following guidelines have been adapted from her work.

Critical incident analysis

(A) What constitutes a critical incident?
- An incident in which you feel your intervention really made a difference in outcome, either directly or indirectly (by helping other staff members).
- An incident that went unusually well.

- An incident in which there was a breakdown (i.e. things did not go as planned).
- An incident that is very ordinary and typical.
- An incident that you think captures the quintessence of what midwifery is all about.
- An incident that was particularly demanding.

(B) What to include in your description of a critical incident
- The context of the incident (e.g. shift, time of day, staff resources).
- A detailed description of what happened.
- Why the incident is 'critical' to you.
- What your concerns were at the time.

(C) What you were thinking about as the incident was taking place
- What you were feeling during and after the incident.
- What, if anything, you found most demanding about the situation.

Within reflective groups, just as in any group work, ground rules need to be set by the participants. A specimen set of rules appears later in this chapter in the section on peer review, but groups will need to determine their own rules. Above all, confidentiality of clients must not be breached; records in reflective diaries and discussions in groups must preserve confidentiality.

Peer review

Peer review may be defined as an assessment of a midwife's action, decisions and practice within a supportive group of like-minded equals. Its aim is to improve and develop practice but also to make explicit the theory which underpins practice. It is only fair to say that peer review within the Centre for Midwifery Practice took many weeks to actually get off the ground! This may have been because for many of the midwives it was an entirely new activity and one which seemed to cause either anxiety or apathy. In the early days of the Centre's activities, it was perceived as not important and as something that could be missed when there was other more pressing work to do. Some of the Canadian MA students studying at Queen Charlotte's College of Health and Science were helpful in suggesting the forms that peer review could take as it is an integral part of independent midwifery practice in British Columbia. They viewed the activity as empowering and team-building as it is directed towards problem solving and the learning achieved through the whole process of review. It is important to state that peer review is not punitive and must be conducted within a safe, supportive and non-threatening environment. When setting it up, we discussed ground rules and agreed on the following, adapted from Kilty & Bond (1992):

- *Confidentiality.* Anything discussed within the group practice's peer review is kept confidential unless the individual midwife decides to share it with a wider audience.
- *Ownership.* Each midwife speaks for herself and not for anyone else.
- *Respect.* Participants must respect each other and individual practices.
- *Autonomy.* Each midwife decides for herself how much to contribute, although there is an expectation that all members of the group practice are involved.
- *Reciprocity.* Each midwife has an equal opportunity to speak and be listened to.
- *Commitment.* Each midwife is expected to attend peer review and to contribute to the group's learning.

Peer review is conducted fortnightly within each group practice and so far, has been facilitated by the lecturer practitioner, although it is hoped that the groups will take over this function in the future. Individual midwives contribute, providing rationale for their actions, and are asked questions by their peers to clarify a situation or to challenge the care given. Thus practice is laid open for scrutiny by colleagues and the midwives are either confirmed in their course of action or enabled to see a different approach.

The discussion often centres on the evidence for practice from research findings using the Cochrane Pregnancy and Childbirth Database. But it is also interesting and worthwhile to explore the practical knowledge of experienced midwives and to uncover the intuitive nature of their decision-making. Thus peer review has largely consisted of the recounting of midwifery care given but has also touched upon obstetric management. As the evaluation of the Centre for Midwifery Practice continues, data will be available on outcomes (such as the epidural rate or the rates of perineal trauma) and this will be incorporated into peer review.

Seminars

Seminars alternate with peer review and are thus held fortnightly on a Wednesday afternoon. Topics have been selected by the midwives and include physiological third stage, the latest Report on Confidential Enquiries into Maternal Deaths (DoH, 1994b), infant resuscitation and intravenous cannulation. Visiting speakers are sometimes invited or the discussion is led by the lecturer practitioner. Other ideas for the future are presentations by the midwives on issues they have explored while studying for degrees or professional qualifications or of journal articles of interest.

Identifying personal development needs

Prior to the commencement of the Centre for Midwifery Practice the midwives who had been provisionally appointed were asked in a questionnaire to review their experience and skills, to identify practice areas in which they wished to gain experience and to highlight issues for discussion as seminar topics. This then formed the basis for discussion during a 30-minute interview with the lecturer practitioner. After this the midwives were asked to complete a personal development plan, which would be reviewed regularly. An example plan is provided in Fig. 3.3. The theory behind this action comes from adult education literature, particularly Knowles' work on learning contracts (1984) and also from an understanding of the UKCC's recommendations (1990) that every practitioner's personal professional profile should contain a self-assessment of educational and developmental needs and a plan to meet them.

It would seem from a small study conducted by the lecturer practitioner with one group practice that the midwives found self-assessment a difficult process, partly because of acknowledging to themselves and others that they had needs in their education and experience and partly because of the timing of the exercise in that many other events and experiences were taking place just prior to the opening of the Centre. The midwives suggested that an individual orientation programme should be worked out well in advance to enable experience in different practice areas and that this should be separate from a personal development plan which is easier to complete once the midwives are actually practising in this new way with an understanding of their own needs.

Even though the midwives experienced some difficulty with identifying their own development needs, they viewed the experience as worthwhile using adjectives such as 'constructive', 'positive' and 'valuable'. It was also evident that some kind of support was vital in the process. Issues to consider are who is best placed to provide this support and should this process be linked to performance review?

Fardell (1991, p. 51) argues that the outcomes of personal action planning should result in 'an improvement in practice or demonstrable professional development'. As a result of planning and achieving their objectives the midwives interviewed expected to become better practitioners – time will tell!

Working side-by-side

There are three ways in which the midwives could be described as

Developmental objective	Proposed actions	Timing
Gain confidence in inserting intravenous cannulae.	Revise anatomy of the arm.	October 1993
	Attend seminar by cannula representative.	November 1993
	Discuss with and observe ODA on delivery suite.	November–December 1993
	Practise under supervision.	January–March 1994
Effective management of my time.	Read literature	
	Discuss with others in group practice ways of working.	
	Attend 1 day course on time management.	March 1994
Gain confidence and skill in home births	Attend study day.	December 1993
	Read appropriate literature.	
	Attend home births as 2nd midwife.	
	Offer home births to women on my caseload and ask experienced midwife to attend as support.	July 1994
Develop effective mentoring/teaching skills.	Complete ENB 997.	March 1994
	Offer to mentor student for 6 months.	March–August 1994
	Read literature on mentoring/reflective practice.	
	Discuss with lecturer practitioner.	
Gain skill in subcuticular suturing	Consult Cochrane Database and read relevant research reports.	January 1994
	Attend seminar on suturing.	February 1994
	Observe experienced midwives/registrars and practise with supervision.	
	Close follow-up of women I've sutured.	
	Discuss at peer review.	

Fig. 3.3   A personal development plan.

working side-by-side and contributing to the peer learning community. The first of these is working side-by-side with a partner. At home births and occasionally in hospital when partners are available to attend births, both sides of the partnership are present and able to observe one another's practice. This has made a significant contribution to learning, particularly when reflection occurs as is encouraged at peer review. Some midwives are particularly skilled at minimizing perineal trauma or at supporting and encouraging women through a long labour and it is helpful to be able to observe their artistry and to use them as role models.

Secondly, the midwives may be described as working side-by-side with the women and families they care for and they form friendships with them. We have encouraged the midwives to seek feedback on their practice from women throughout their care, but particularly after labour, asking questions such as 'was there anything I did which was particularly helpful/unhelpful?'

An area of concern raised by one group practice at peer review described the potential difficulty that midwives may experience in making appropriate decisions when the women they care for become friends and whether or not this might 'cloud' their judgement. Many of the midwives have also found difficulty in saying goodbye and discharging women from their care. We have used Campbell's notion of skilled companionship (1984) and his image of a journey where companionship arises from a chance meeting and is ended when the journey is completed. Campbell describes the good companion as someone who 'shares freely, but does not impose, allowing others to make their own journey' (p. 49) – a beautiful description of midwifery care. Although companionship may be costly and demanding (particularly when called at 2 AM on a winter's night), it is a limited commitment where woman and midwife are together for a while and then part, allowing each other to journey on.

Thirdly, on occasions the midwives work side-by-side with the lecturer practitioner. This is usually when the lecturer practitioner needs the help of a second midwife at a home birth but may also be when midwives request her to work with them for a morning to assess their practice for the clinical component of modules they may be undertaking. Time is always given to reflecting on the experience with a view to gaining new knowledge and insight.

Excellence in practice

What is the nature of midwifery practice encouraged in the Centre? We have already mentioned artistry in describing skilled midwifery practice. Schön (1991) defines artistry as the competence by which practitioners handle the indeterminate zones of practice that present messy, confusing problems which at times defy technical solution. Schön also describes artistry as an exercise of intelligence, a kind of knowing which is rigorous in its own terms.

Few will forget Jayne Torvill and Christopher Dean's gold medal performance in the 1985 Olympic ice dancing competition – their breathtakingly beautiful performance to the haunting music of Ravel's *Bolero* and their maximum 6.0 score from all nine judges for artistic impression. Yet such a sensitive and magical interpretation was based upon hours and hours of listening to the music, many weeks of careful, painstaking choreography and months and months of rigorous practice and training.

The midwife who uses artistry in her practice will combine and hold in harmony her intellectual, personal and practical skills to provide excellence in her care. Artistry in practice is dependent upon a culture which welcomes creativity and innovation and which encourages enquiry, debate and learning. Benner (1984) writes of the knowledge embedded in the practice of experts which really amounts to artistry. Through peer review, reflection and working side-by-side we hope that this knowledge will be unearthed and made available to midwives.

To go further in our understanding of the nature of practice, James & Clarke's model of collaborative practice (1993) strikes a chord with our experience in the Centre for Midwifery Practice. They identify five elements or 'commitments' which interlink and provide the framework for their model:

(1) *A commitment to the development of theory.* We have already described the purpose of theory and the importance of generating theory from practice in developing a body of midwifery knowledge. James & Clarke assert that in collaborative practice there must be a commitment to formulate one's own theory of practice which needs to be constantly reviewed, refined and developed.
(2) *A commitment to development through reflective practice.* A significant element of collaborative practice is learning from experience through reflection and we have described ways of encouraging this through different learning activities.
(3) *A commitment to continuous improvement.* The commitment to continuous improvement is an integral part of the Centre with its emphasis on professional and personal development and contribution to the peer learning community.
(4) *A commitment to autonomy.* James & Clarke describe this element as individuals 'knowing and asserting their own value and that of their clients and colleagues' (p. 6). The Centre encourages midwives to practice within the full extent of their role and to re-discover the worth of midwifery but also to recognize the boundaries of midwifery practice.

(5) *A commitment to collaboration*. 'Essentially, collaboration is working in association with others, or in conjunction with them. It means working separately and independently but with similar understanding of, and commitment to, similar values and goals' (James & Clarke, 1993, p. 7). This succinctly describes the nature of practice within the Centre and its promotion of a peer learning community with its organization into partnerships and group practices.

Conclusion

The midwifery profession currently seeks to define the body of knowledge which underpins its practice and on which its claim to autonomy rests (Alexander, *et al.*, 1990). Benner (1984) acknowledges that for some expert practitioners, knowledge is tacit, evident to all, but difficult to articulate and quantify. Schön (1991) examines the difficulties of recognizing and encouraging artistry in practice and professional education and Jarvis (1987) stresses the need to bridge the chasm between systematic, scientific knowledge and competent clinical practice.

Within this chapter, we have suggested that scholarship in midwifery depends on putting art into practice by identifying and articulating the hallmarks of the effective practitioner. We have offered ways of encouraging an enquiring atmosphere in which scholarship is seen as a necessary, worthwhile and collaborative pursuit. We have considered how midwives can be enabled in their own development, recognizing their professional development needs and formulating plans to meet them. Developing scholarship in practice has not been presented as an easy task, but neither is it impossible. As midwives act in their roles as 'skilled companions' to women, they need to be valued, supported and enabled to think in new ways. The strategies we have described in this chapter may address this important issue.

Chapter 4
The Emancipated Doctor:
A New Relationship between
Midwife and Obstetrician

Introduction

Much of this book is about developing the role of the midwife. But we should remember that even with increased professional autonomy midwives and doctors will continue to work together as colleagues, and still often as part of a team. In this chapter we talk about ways in which the working relationship between midwives and doctors might change, and the effect that that change might have. Thoughtful redefinition of the respective roles of doctor and midwife will be an important part of the change within the maternity services. Before defining any event anew, it is necessary to look into the past to see whether there is a precedent. A knowledge of history is vitally important for us all as it is because of what has gone before that we react in the way that we do in the present.

Obstetrics in the UK was born in the mid eighteenth century. A small hospital for the care of women in childbirth (Queen Charlotte's) opened in London. William Smellie began his practice as 'man midwife' in Lanarkshire, Scotland. He developed a reputation for manual dexterity in being able to deliver women who had obstructed labour and for whom their attending midwives could do no more. A midwife to obstetrician referral pattern had started. On moving to London his reputation as an obstetrician and teacher increased and in 1752 his famous *Treatise on the Theory and Practice of Midwifery* was published. In this volume he described his obstetrical methods with great clarity and detail including events such as type 2 decelerations of the fetal heart during labour. As a good teacher he attracted pupils who were then taught as apprentices and so obstetric practice started in the UK. Use of forceps as a method of helping certain deliveries, developed both in the UK and France at this time. They were being used by their pioneers to help with prolonged and obstructed labour and so obstetricians developed the reputation for, and the right to, operative vaginal delivery. Despite the dexterity required for these manoeuvres, obstetricians were still essentially physicians while gynaecological surgery was carried out by general surgeons. Gradually obstetrics and gynaecology came together as

47

specialities and by the late nineteenth and early twentieth centuries, the discipline of obstetrics and gynaecology had developed and was then firmly in the surgical camp.

However, it was not until 1929 that the Royal College of Obstetricians and Gynaecologists was set up, thereby moving obstetrics and gynaecology out of the surgical camp and establishing it as a speciality in its own right. During the evolution of obstetrics and gynaecology as a specialty most women were cared for entirely by midwives and general practitioners working on an equal footing with each other and they were delivered in their own homes. A small but increasing number of the complications of pregnancy and labour were being cared for in obstetrical units, attached to the teaching hospitals that were springing up in the nineteenth and early twentieth centuries.

Historical influences

Move to hospital-based care

Major changes took place as a result of World War II. The advent of antibiotics meant that obstetrical units did not have to be separated from other specialities because of the risk of infection. The development of blood transfusion and the Flying Squad led to greater emphasis being placed on the association between hospital care and safety. Midwives were again transferring patients from their care at home to obstetricians in hospitals when things went wrong. Domiciliary midwifery declined rapidly during the 1950s and 1960s and was replaced by confinement in hospitals or small general practitioner-run maternity units in cottage hospitals or attached to District General hospitals. In hospital practice, the obstetrician was the dominant partner, while midwives gradually assumed the roles of assistants to the obstetrician and of nurse, despite the fact that they personally conducted about 70% of deliveries. This was in contrast to the state of affairs in general practitioner units and in domiciliary practice where the role of the midwife was equal to and complemented that of the doctor.

Changing role of general practitioners

General practitioners, initially the sole providers of obstetric care for all mothers other than those with a clearly defined complication, became increasingly sidelined in maternity care. Starting at a time of low morale in the 1950s and early 1960s, general practitioners were reduced to working with the consolation prize of antenatal observations and occasional referral.

There was a brief attempt during the late 1970s at redressing the balance in the form of general practitioner unit care, in which general practitioners and community midwives supervised antenatal care together, and contracted to provide intrapartum care within the hospital environment. They provided continuity of care in the relative safety of a designated suite within the hospital where, for emergencies, immediate senior obstetric expertise was at hand.

But most general practitioners in the 1970s and 1980s, were providing antenatal care only (with the occasional unintentional home delivery) working alongside a lone and sometimes part-time community midwife. They shared the responsibility of preparing the mother for childbirth, and the concern for her and her family's well-being afterwards. Many chose not to practise intra partum obstetrics, although in the event of a home delivery, general practitioner and midwife would attend quickly and together, to provide all the care and expertise at their command.

Growing power of obstetricians

With increasing emphasis on the use of technology as a means to ensure the safety of mother and baby, obstetric units were seen as the best place to have a baby and the obstetricians' power grew. This reached its peak in the mid 1970s when induction of labour was deemed by obstetricians as the appropriate way to start labour in up to 45% of women in many units and the automatic infusion of syntocinon by a self-regulating pump (Cardiff Pump) was the ultimate in technology. Women had become trapped by the technology which obstetricians enjoyed using as it gave them more control over events and was a substitute for scientific thinking about the problems of obstetrics. There was little or no attention given to the emotional needs of the patients.

The patient rebellion

Eventually the patients themselves rebelled and obstetricians were forced to re-think their clinical practice and their attitudes. By the late 1970s and early 1980s changes such as more homely wards, early discharge and a more flexible approach to labour were becoming more common. It became normal practice to accept partners in labour wards. However, there was not much change in the role of the midwife for some time.

The present

Stereotypes of obstetrician and midwife

Let us look at the stereotypical roles of obstetrician and midwife at present on the basis of who does what, and why. The obstetricians book the patient, do all the antenatal checks, make all decisions concerning management of pregnancy and labour if appropriate and deal with any problems that may occur. The obstetrician has little if anything to do with labour.

The midwife, on the other hand, talks to the patient, explains things and issues certificates. Once the patient is admitted in labour the midwife is suddenly in charge and responsible for reporting any abnormalities. It is only with shared care that the midwife may have a continuing role, but it is unlikely to be the same midwife. The disadvantages to the patient are lack of continuity of care and lack of security and confidence. The advantage is that she will get prompt obstetrical intervention if things go wrong. The majority therefore pay a potential price for the benefit of a minority.

The role of the midwife in practice

What can happen in practice? This will depend on personalities, and personal relationships. Here are some examples. One of us had the following experience:

'On my first night of obstetrics in a small isolated maternity unit, I was summoned at 2.30 AM to a case of severe abruption which I had never dealt with before. I sleepily looked in a text book but after a few minutes realized I wasn't taking in what I was trying to read and that I had better get to the labour ward. Fortunately the sister in charge was very experienced, and had everything ready. She quietly guided me step-by-step as we went along. This was a wonderful educational experience for me and good management for the patient. In the same hospital I was on call for two weeks continuously. The same sister used to encourage me to go out for a few hours once or twice a week (unofficially). While away, she would happily do forcep deliveries if necessary and had undoubtedly done very many more forcep deliveries than I would ever have a chance to do in the immediate future. Manual skills need not be the sole right of the obstetrician and particularly very junior ones.'

A second example occurred in a teaching hospital's busy antenatal clinic. Two doctors were away in the labour ward and patients were waiting for a long time. There were two rooms empty and the sister in charge said, 'we can't find another doctor'. There were three trained midwives in the clinic doing clerical duties when the suggestion was made that one or more of them might see patients. It was rejected as not being possible.

A third example occurred one day when a general practitioner was having morning coffee. A telephone call from a harassed and breathless man came through, 'my daughter is having a baby'. The general practitioner absentmindedly muttered congratulations and continued to drink his coffee. The penny slowly dropped: 'Where is your daughter?' and the exasperated reply came back, 'On the landing upstairs'. At this point the midwife arrived on cue to start the antenatal clinic at the surgery. It took very little time for both general practitioner and midwife to reach the mother-to-be, waters broken, late in second stage and pushing, indeed on the carpet of the landing upstairs. A little boy was born, to the absolute incredulity of the girl's father. This concealed pregnancy was delivered successfully helped by the confidence of a team midwife accompanied by the girl's surprised general practitioner.

In the first instance the midwife was experienced, competent, confident and enjoyed her job. In the second case the midwives had lost their confidence in practising their skills. In the third case the midwife already working in the community, but trained in intra partum obstetrics, was able to meet an unexpected situation with adroitness and expertise.

New guidelines for practice

Obstetric practice has over the last 30–40 years intentionally or unintentionally reduced the role of the midwife to that of an assistant, but one that is still supposed to carry out 80% of deliveries competently and take responsibility for them. In caring for the pregnant woman three groups of professionals are involved, namely midwife, obstetrician and general practitioner. All are agreed that they want the best care for mothers and babies. We all have a different concept of what that care involves and how it should be delivered. The present care lacks continuity and security for the mother because these cannot be met by obstetricians alone and the midwife lacks an appropriate role. The Royal Colleges of the three professional groups have recently come together and made jointly a number of important statements.

Some of these statements are:

'(1) There should be a clear coherent policy at national level that allows for the provision of comprehensive and co-ordinated services at a local level.
(2) Service provision should respond to change and knowledge as well as social needs.
(3) Women should receive highly personalized care.
(4) There should be continuity of care, with good communications between different groups or individuals involved.
(5) The emotional comfort of women is as important as their physical well being.'

(RCOG, RCM, RCGP, 1992)

The Royal Colleges felt that these aims could be best met by midwives having an identifiable caseload and being enabled as far as possible to develop a one-to-one relationship with their clients. These views were shared by the Select Committee of the House of Commons in the Winterton Report (1992). This would give back to the midwife the professional responsibility that has been lost during the last half century. The Cumberlege Report (1993), has further reinforced the case to reinstate the role of midwife as autonomous practitioner. These guidelines cannot be ignored as they are what pregnant women want and what midwives want. If they are to be implemented, we will be moving back towards midwives and doctors working as equals.

The changing role of the midwife

The changes that we are currently seeing are a continuation of the events described but they have taken some time to come about. This is because the woman's need for better care has taken time to be realized. Better care comprises more continuity, more emotional security and more flexibility but without compromising the medical safety. This is not easy to achieve in a medically dominated system. But the focus is beginning to change. The emphasis is now on the midwife, the general practitioner and most importantly the patient, now regarded more appropriately, as a client.

Changing the role of the midwife in practice

The Kidlington Team

Changes can more readily take place in general practice when the respected parties are less entrenched. The last five years have seen major changes in the provision of antenatal care in the community. Here in Kidlington the work of our single part-time community midwife has been transformed by the introduction of team midwifery. In 1989 her workload was widened in effect to include once again intrapartum obstetrics. She was joined by five full-time hospital midwives who came to work alongside her in the community. One of us was involved in this early development which drew national attention, and was an example for others to follow. Community care was the underlying philosophy and the mother was made central to the decision-making processes involved in pregnancy and childbirth.

The introduction of change in the context of general practice is almost always fraught. The concept of team midwifery was both welcomed and reviled by differing team members. Certainly part of the problem was the speed of the changes or timescale over which the general practitioners were expected to react. Eventually we had midwives allocated to each of the doctors involved and, antenatal, intrapartum and postnatal care was assured for the 250 women, in this population of about 14 000 who give birth each year.

Who does what: the impact of the midwifery team on care

In general practice the change in the working ways of the midwives produced changes in obstetric care. The presence of the midwifery team, by its size, has increased the profile of the care of pregnant women in the practice. There has been a move away from hospital-based care, to general practice 'medical centre' orientated care, and towards care of the pregnant women in the home. The first booking session with the woman is conducted by a team midwife in the home. Taking up to an hour, it is likely that it alters the balance of power in the relationship in favour of the pregnant woman: the carer ventures into her territory. Similarly, towards the end of pregnancy, the labour talk conducted at home emphasizes the desire to give back to the woman as far as possible control over her mode of delivery.

This investment of time in the home redresses the balance of power away from the hospital and general practitioner, via the midwife to the mother. There is some evidence (Watson, 1990) that it may influence the use of analgesia in labour and possibly the occurrence of intervention. From the point of view of setting the mother centre stage in maternity care, it is good. But it leaves some concern in the minds of general practitioners as the centre of control of their client's obstetric care moves away from them. This has also made general practitioners jealous of their role as family doctors. Nursing their loss of privilege with the mother, sidelined, they re-examine their own roles.

Supporting colleagues

The changes in community care obstetrics have brought a greater awareness of the importance of a joint approach to problem solving. The presence of the midwifery team at primary health care team meetings has emphasized the stature and importance of maternity care in the community, but it has also brought with it tensions. It is necessary to demonstrate open support and care for one another's colleagues if the mother's needs are to be met; to share concerns with the relevant team members and advise and counsel in the face of adversity. Health visitors play an important part in the welfare of the family and their involvement antenatally is vital if anticipatory care is to be offered. The health visitor, herself a trained nurse, will often be witness to a delayed impact of the problems of pregnancy and subsequent puerperal difficulties both physical and emotional.

The diversity of the personalities involved in team midwifery has made it more difficult, but perhaps more important than ever, to maintain a good professional relationship between health visitors and midwives and general practitioners. The shared experience of the different professionals can shed light on the needs of individual mothers. It is endlessly fascinating to witness at a big primary health care team meeting the wealth of information that comes out, if sought, and the light it brings to bear on a family with problems in pregnancy. Mothers are quite particular about with whom they are prepared to share confidences, and these confidences in turn need to be treated with great delicacy and skill if they are to be used to her best advantage.

Relationship between general practitioner and midwife in developing the practice

It is apparent that responsibility in antenatal care is going to move away from general practitioners towards the midwife, with the mother remaining central to all concerns. One of the fears of general practitioners is loss of contact with the woman at an important, usually happy and sometimes traumatic, but always life changing time in her life. Midwives now rightly dominate normal pregnancy; the general practioner misses out. With this loss of involvement goes perhaps something of the satisfaction of practising family medicine. The general practitioner misses the excitement of childbirth and by contrast continues the plodding, caring, involvement with the ordinary events in a woman's life and that of her family. Few other countries in the world can match the British general practitioner's complete commitment to the family, witnessing the growth and development of two, three and sometimes even more generations in a working lifetime. Special knowledge about patients is jealously guarded and yet the wisdom and knowledge of the general practitioner is never more needed than during pregnancy when he or she can provide the context of a women's hopes, fears and concerns.

Sometimes working with team midwives can dissipate that sharing. In order to ensure adequate transfer of information in both directions, it has become more important than ever to continue talking together, negotiating, compromising, informing and helping.

Part of this sharing and concern for the mother can be assured by taking care of the practical aspects of the organization of maternity care; not always easy in a busy health centre. To organize even the basic logistical chores of ensuring a consulting room with a computer for both midwife and general practitioner, and to run the two simultaneously with three other surgeries, can be time consuming and tricky, requiring skills in person management as well as a logical mind. The professionals concerned, while battling for the foreground, must always keep in mind that they are only one part of a bigger team, all of whom are working to better the lives and well-being of childbearing women.

Respective roles of the general practitioner, the midwife and the obstetrician

In the future the general practitioner's role is going to alter in two significant ways. The first is in the clinical area of obstetric management. In the future, obstetric care will be streamed from the outset into high and low risk pregnancies, based on a combination of medical and obstetric criteria examined jointly by both midwife and general practitioner. High risk pregnancies will remain in the province of the hospital specialists, with general practioner and midwife complementing hospital care. Low risk pregnancies will be judged from booking and their management will become much more individually suited to each pregnant woman's need.

The rigid periods of review used at present (four weekly interval up to 28 weeks; two weekly until 36, then weekly thereafter) will be abandoned in favour of more goal-oriented visits (Hall, *et al.*, 1985; RCOG, 1982) combining thorough antenatal screening. The schedule might consist of bloods at 16 weeks, a fetal anomaly scan at 19 weeks and growth checks at 26 weeks. Weighing will be confined to an accurate body mass index estimation at booking. Also, the antenatal period will be a time when the woman's midwife/midwives will get to know her. The general practitioner will be less involved with the obstetric care per se and more involved in checking aspects of the family as a whole; paediatric involvement will become particularly important. It is likely that discharge from hospital within 24 hours will become more frequent and that the general practitioner will begin the contract for child health care and immunization with the initial postnatal check of the baby. The midwife will have very much greater influence over the pregnancy, working with colleagues to generate an antenatal plan tailored to the individual woman's needs. Antenatal care will become essentially the responsiblity of the midwife again, for the majority of women.

In Britain the second way in which the general practitioner's role will change is in taking over financial administration of community care obstetrics. Because of reforms in the NHS there is a great shift of financial emphasis away from hospital-based medicine to community care, and one way this is being arranged is by giving general practioners their own community care budgets to manage. It seems likely that eventually this will include the process of buying not just the community care services of the district nurses and mental health team, but also those of the midwives. It is inevitable that there will be a redress of the balance of power in the obstetric care of the community back from the midwifery led team to the purchasing of general practitioners as they negotiate the quality of care that will be offered. Such a change will bring with it great demands on the quality of leadership of both doctors and midwives, requiring that the need to enshrine the principles of continuity, effectiveness and accessibility is recognized.

Role of the obstetrician

Leadership in redefining roles

Given the midwife's current role, some, perhaps most, of the leadership in trying to attain a meeting of minds must come from the medical staff. Failure to give this lead will put midwives on the defensive, with all the barriers that that throws up. Positive relationships between general practitioners, obstetricians and midwives are crucial if amicable team-work is to provide the right atmosphere in which to deliver good care. This means that the doctor should no longer be seen as the expert, with the midwife in an inferior role. Rather, the relationship should be one of two equals but with each having certain skills that are complementary to those of the other.

The obstetrician has at present a monopoly on the skills for operative delivery, but there is no reason why this needs to be the case. Midwives with appropriate expertise and training could be just as able as a doctor to use a Ventouse vacuum extractor or deliver a breech. The obstetrician will always be the one who will wield the knife, by virtue of having a theoretical degree in surgery. Again the obstetrician will have a greater knowledge of general medicine and pathology by virtue of a medical training compared with midwifery training. This makes the obstetrician the appropriate person to deal with the medical problems of pregnant women and the problems of pregnancy, such as pre-eclampsia, that require a knowledge of general medicine.

The midwife, who is dealing with normal pregnancy and labour and who is trained to recognize the abnormal without necessarily managing it, is the best person to look after the majority of pregnant women. This role has many advantages. It allows the midwife to go into the community, to arrange for more flexibly timed clinics, to discuss more freely the anxieties of a pregnant woman, and to spend the extra time that good continuous care requires. The midwife should be the one with the best skills in conducting normal labour and delivery and should be free from attending to other duties so as to be able to be present throughout labour. Handing over to someone else in the middle of labour, when the patient is at her most vulnerable physically and emotionally, is not the best care – but with the present rigid hospital system, it is inevitable.

To facilitate continuity of care with the patient and the midwife being the key players a system of one-to-one midwifery care has been set up within the Centre for Midwifery Practice in the Queen Charlotte's and

Hammersmith Maternity Service, The Hammersmith Hospitals Trust. This is a demonstration study based on a limited geographical area and is currently being evaluated both clinically and financially. Three teams of six midwives, working in pairs, are attempting to provide full midwifery care to the patients allotted to them. Patients are categorized according to low and high risk. For the low risk patients the midwife is the leading professional while the high risk patients are looked after in the conventional hospital-based manner by obstetricians. The midwives are on call in pairs, carry mobile telephones and drive their own cars. They provide patients with antenatal care, in the home, in the general practitioner's surgery or in hospital clinics, whichever is the most convenient, and they are responsible for this as well as delivering the patient and providing the postnatal care. Formal visits to hospital are limited to three, namely at booking, at 28 weeks and at 41 weeks. It is the responsibility of the midwife to seek appropriate help at other times if things go wrong.

This approach is consistent with proposals put forward in the Cumberlege Report (1993) that women should have a named midwife and so more personal care. However, these proposals have raised people's expectations very considerably and even with a programme as outlined above there are occasions when both members of the pair are otherwise occupied and the patient has to see a third member of the group. Nevertheless the approach is consistent with what patients want and expect and is a form of practice that is more satisfying for the midwives, giving them back their autonomy and sense of independence which has been lost over the past 30 years. We hope that the evaluation, which is being carried out by an independent group of experts, will be favourable and that the project can be extended to cover all of our practice.

In the meantime it is worth recording potential problems. Firstly the planning period was more than one year. This apparently long time was necessary to get the concept across to the medical staff and to the midwives, to recruit senior staff to run the project, to draw up protocols for clinical care and get these agreed with the medical staff, to recruit the evaluation group and to draw up questionnaires and finally to get the agreement and support of the local general practitioners. We have been successful in these aims but it has taken time.

Recruitment of midwives to work on an on-call basis with one partner was thought to be a potential problem but did not prove to be one. The concept of working as a professional with continuous responsibility rather than on a shift system has been welcomed. How this arrangement will stand the test of time remains to be seen, however, but so far so good. There are potential conflicts between, on the one hand, these midwives working in one particular way and, on the other hand, the hospital-based midwives working conventional shift patterns. Again, with communication between both groups clarifying their respective roles these problems can be resolved quite easily. The project and its rigorous evaluation has had considerable support from the Regional Health Authority.

Training of doctors

The importance of midwives as teachers both of medical students and of senior house officers has also begun to be recognized at last. The unenviable position of senior house officers (SHOs) having extensive responsibility on the delivery suite but often skills far inferior to those of the senior midwife working with them is now being addressed. The RCOG/RCGP working party (1992) recommends a contribution by midwives to the training programme for SHOs, many of whom will become general practitioners. Midwives should be encouraged to teach SHOs normal obstetric practices while the role of the SHO should be to provide liaison between midwife, registrar and consultant, as well as the assessment of the management of obstetric abnormalities. Ideally SHOs should be keeping log books of their experience, which should be examined bi-monthly by their consultant or teaching registrar. Attendance at antenatal and postnatal clinics should become part of the essential experience of the obstetric SHO training, together with provision of family planning training. Admission to the obstetric list in general practice and or progression on to the specialist ladder of obstetrics itself would as ever be governed by the procedure of examinations. It is vital if this kind of training programme is to succeed that senior midwives and doctors develop relationships fitting to this situation, ensuring that knowledge is passed on and that the patient has the care she needs and deserves.

Conclusion

We need to create the environment in which both midwife and doctor can function most effectively and can provide the mother with optimum care. This means breaking down our rigid hierarchical structure, defining our respective roles and determining proper referral patterns. If this can be done, the obstetrician, the midwife and the general practitioner can work together harmoniously, heeding the words of their respective Royal Colleges. The care received by pregnant women will improve. The lead in this process should come from obstetricians. They must not see change as a diminution of their role, but as a redefinition that allows them to do what they are trained to do in a more satisfactory and fulfilling way.

Chapter 5
Who is Left Holding the Baby?
Meeting the Challenge of the
Winterton Report

Awaiting the Winterton Report

The summer of 1991 was an exciting time for midwives. The House of Commons Select Committee Enquiry into Maternity Services was moving fast. Evidence had been taken from professional and consumer groups and from individuals.

The Committee had decided to 'make normal birth of healthy babies to healthy women the starting point and focus' of their enquiry. Assuming high significance in their discussions was the conviction that women had the right to 'a life-enhancing start to their family life'.

The evidence presented to the Committee had convinced members of 'the desire of women for the provision of continuity of care and carer throughout pregnancy and childbirth' and that the majority of women receiving maternity care 'regard midwives as the best placed and equipped to provide this' (Winterton Report 1992). By late summer it was becoming apparent that the Committee was likely to recommend wide sweeping changes in the existing patterns of midwifery care and that many of the aspirations of the midwifery profession were assuming reality. But there were a considerable number of obstacles to be overcome if these exciting possibilities were to be achieved.

Obstacles to change

Patterns of maternity care and midwifery work

Although three groups of health care professionals – midwives, general practitioners and obstetricians – had jointly provided maternity care, the way that care had evolved within the National Health Service (NHS) had produced a hierarchical, medical model of care. This had the effect of reducing the role and status of midwives from professional colleagues to that of a 'secondary' or 'assistant' professional even though they took responsibility for delivering about 70% of all babies, and the management of postnatal care. The impetus for these subtle and unplanned changes came from the publication of the Peel Report (1970), and the reorganization of the NHS in 1974. Before that time babies were born

59

either at home, under the care of the domiciliary midwife employed by the local authority, or in a general practitioner-run maternity unit, or in a NHS run hospital where women were booked under the care of doctors, and midwives worked under their direction. When the NHS was reorganized in 1974, all maternity care came under the jurisdiction of the NHS. From that time, numbers of home deliveries reduced until they were almost unknown and reorganization of local services combined with ill-founded arguments against the safety and cost-effectiveness of general practitioner maternity units (Tew, 1990, Klein *et al.*, 1983) led to their widespread demise.

Effects of the adoption of the 'medical' model for maternity care

Services were increasingly organized on a medical or sickness model. The most common pattern of care was for a pregnant woman to be referred by her general practitioner to an obstetrician in order to obtain a hospital bed for the birth of her baby. These referrals of healthy women to antenatal clinics followed the same pattern as those for medical or surgical out-patients. Despite the fact that midwives took the responsibility for delivering about 70% of all babies, adopting the medical model of care led to erosion of the autonomy of the midwife as practitioner, anomalies in the function and role of midwives and junior doctors working in hospitals and duplication of effort between community midwives and general practitioners.

The way that midwifery work was organized also created problems. In the hospital the work of midwives revolved around shifts and rotas in wards and departments, and there was often a hierarchical approach to allocating work, which did not make the best use of the skills and experience of midwives. This was a particular problem for midwives who wished to work part-time. Although community midwives had more freedom in managing their work, this was largely restrained by the number of antenatal clinics and the demands of providing postnatal care to women returned home earlier in the puerperium. The opportunities for delivering babies diminished as home and general practitioner unit deliveries reduced, and the practice of general practitioner attachment, and the lack of any means of assessing or controlling workload frequently led to unequal allocation of work. In an effort to reduce these effects a number of systems such as domino schemes, and team midwifery were developed. These were designed to improve continuity of care to mothers and to maintain the skills of midwives, but they were frequently hampered by fixed work patterns related to rotas, shifts and a $37\frac{1}{2}$ hour working week, and the attitude of some managers did not help (Flint & Poulengeris 1987). Frustration with the inability to practise fully as a midwife within the NHS had led some midwives to adopt independent practice.

Resistance to change

It was anticipated that there might be resistance to the proposed changes from some obstetricians and general practitioners, most of whose practice had been within the existing service, and who might combine reluctance to change with doubts about the ability of the midwifery profession to meet the proposed patterns of care. It was also likely that many midwives who had trained and practised within the current system might be daunted by the demands of practitioner-based work.

Managing the change

Although there were a number of pioneering models of midwifery-led care, such as the Know Your Midwife scheme (Flint, 1987), and the establishment of midwifery run sectors within a large teaching hospital (Morris-Thompson, 1993) there was no universally adopted model. Those which had been developed depended largely upon local agreements and co-operation of general practitioners and obstetricians. In other areas this degree of harmony and co-operation had not been forthcoming. Without a clear strategy, it might be difficult to demonstrate the feasibility of midwifery-led care and its potential benefits and cost implications. This was particularly important in view of the need to work within the many restrictions of finance, and the importance of maintaining current services whilst developing the new patterns of care. Defining a vision for the future is a crucial part of initiating and managing change. As one of the acknowledged experts on organizational management remarked, 'The management of the future has to go hand in hand with the responsibility for the present' (Handy, 1985 p. 373). Achieving major changes in the role and status of midwives would be no easy task.

Problems in the NHS as a whole

The many changes affecting the NHS as a whole, meant that it was not a good time to impose any further change. The implementation of the Government's NHS strategy, *Working for Patients* (DoH, 1989) had led to a new concept of hospitals, community services and health authorities working as provider and purchaser units. The impetus for provider units to become independent NHS Trusts had created further upheaval and uncertainty in the service as a whole. The dearth of methods for assessing workload and workforce requirements (Ball, 1993) meant that midwifery managers had very little information with which to plan or present a viable strategy for development, and the rapid change to a business-oriented culture was creating a situation in which vague aspirations for change, or the possibility of increased costs in a service would not be taken seriously.

Taking the initiative in devising a strategy

Given these formidable problems, there was concern that the opportunities which were expected to be provided by the recommendations of the Select Committee, might be lost, not because of any lack of skill or commitment, but because of the many problems associated with managing change in a complex and already pressurized health service. Managing change requires a clear vision of the future and its benefits, combined with well thought out strategies for its achievement.

Debating the issues

In response to this concern, a group of senior midwives met together in the autumn of 1991 in order to debate the issues and if possible devise a strategy for change and a model of practice which might provide the way forward. The five midwives who met together did so on their own initiative. As a team they combined wide experience in developing woman-centred care, team midwifery, independent midwifery, workload, workforce and quality assessment methods, together with experience in education, management and professional matters.

Taking the initiative

It was intended that the strategy which emerged should be presented as soon as possible after the publication of the Winterton Report in order to:

- Promote a positive debate among all those concerned with the delivery of maternity services.
- Stifle the voices of those who would claim that the expected recommendations were unrealistic.
- Give support to midwifery managers who would have the responsibility of responding to the Report's recommendations.

Any strategy would need to be viable within the context of:

- The available midwifery skills;
- Close working relationships with obstetricians and general practitioners;
- Fulfilling consumer demands;
- Fitting the new purchaser/provider contracts.

Secondly, the timing was held to be crucial. Past experience following the publication of an earlier report on maternity care (Short Report, 1980) had shown that waiting for 'others' to take action had meant that initiatives were lost. The midwifery profession needed to show itself capable of redirecting its practice and of managing the complex changes in professional relationships and service delivery which responding to the expected recommendations would entail. Therefore it was planned to publish the resulting strategy to coincide with the publication of the Winterton Report and to present it at two national conferences, as soon as possible afterwards.

Producing a strategy for action: who's left holding the baby?

The aims of the meetings

The terms of reference were defined as:

'To be creative in defining the type of organisation of midwifery service which would meet consumer expectations and make the most effective use of midwives' resources and reduce duplication of effort in the maternity service as a whole.

To produce an operational framework which would help midwifery managers to implement change in line with the expected recommendations from the Select Committee, and enable midwives at different levels of experience and at different stages of their careers to practise effectively, but not necessarily within the present organisation of midwifery work.'

Ball, *et al.*, 1992

There were a number of questions to be addressed:

- How would the patterns of midwifery work be changed to enable a flexible woman-centred service to become a reality?
- What framework for professional development would enable midwives to adopt different aspects of work at different stages of their careers, especially during times when family commitments took priority over professional ones.

The response to these questions led to a set of proposals which fell into three main areas:

- Consumer choice and the principle of the primary provider;
- Changes in the management and organization of care;
- Changes in the career paths of midwives.

Consumer choice and the principle of the primary provider

There were two related issues: the high degree of consumer discontent with the way maternity care was fragmented, especially around professional demarcation lines; and the need to free midwives from staffing the hospital or community services to 'staffing the women' (Page; House of Commons Report, 1992, p. 979).

Consumer choice

There was some doubt that women had any real choice in their care. Apart from a few remaining home or general practitioner unit deliveries, the usual pattern was for all women to be referred by their general practitioner to an obstetrician, even though the pregnancy and birth of the baby were expected to be normal. Many women first saw a midwife either in the general practitioner's surgery or in the hospital antenatal clinic, where they might be seen as 'secondary' to the main professional, i.e. the general practitioner or the obstetrician and/or his junior staff. There was need to establish the midwife as an equal practitioner in normal pregnancy care. There were also problems when the consumer was passed from the care of one practitioner to another. Not only did this make for difficulties in establishing and maintaining a trusting relationship between the consumer and her carers, but it was also particularly difficult when the woman needed emergency care.

There was need for one professional to be identified as the person who took the main responsibility for planning and co-ordinating the woman's care throughout the pregnancy, birth and the puerperium. This person was defined within the strategy as the *primary provider*. The later Cumberlege Report (1993) uses the term *lead professional* to describe this role.

The strategy recommended that consumers should be able to make an informed choice about their preferred pattern of care. This would be led by a *primary provider* who might be a midwife, a general practitioner with specialist knowledge and interest in normal maternity care, or a consultant obstetrician. The function of primary providers and their continuing responsibility for the care of their clients was defined as follows:

'In all cases, the primary provider will be responsible for ensuring the necessary care and support throughout pregnancy, labour and the post-natal period, providing a 24 hour service to clients. Where transfer in an emergency is needed, the primary provider should accompany the client and continue to provide support in liaison with the consultant obstetrician. Health care purchasers would arrange contracts between groups or individual primary care providers as needed by their population.'

(Ball, *et al.*, 1992)

Shifting the emphasis of care

Establishing the concept of the primary provider would shift the emphasis in providing maternity care, making normal pregnancy the basis for care management, and would cause the development of a different set of relationships between the professionals involved. In the majority of cases the primary provider would be a midwife or general practitioner. If problems arose later in the pregnancy or labour, the client would be referred to an obstetrician for expert care and transferred back to the primary provider once the crisis had been resolved. Where problems existed or were anticipated at the beginning of the pregnancy, or where the client preferred, the first choice would be an obstetrician. If midwives were to be able to fulfil the role of primary provider they would need to have direct access to laboratory services, sonar scan, midwifery beds etc. This was recognized in the later recommendations of the Winterton Report (1992) which are shown in Fig. 5.1.

Working relationships between care providers

There are a number of ways in which midwives could fulfil the role of primary care provider. In order to explore these it is necessary to make distinctions between maternity care and midwifery care. Maternity care can be defined as the oversight and responsibility for providing care as described above. This might include ensuring that a client is referred to

---

We recommend that:

- The status of midwives as professionals is acknowledged in their terms of employment ... on the presumption that they have the right to develop and audit their own professional standards.
- We should move as rapidly as possible towards a situation in which midwives have their own caseload and take full responsibility for the women under their care.
- Midwives be given the opportunity to establish and run midwife-managed maternity units within and outside hospitals.
- The right of midwives to admit women to NHS hospitals should be made explicit.

Fig. 5.1 Recommendations regarding midwifery practice. (Winterton Report, vol. I, p. XCVIII, 1992.)

an obstetrician as required. It also includes ensuring that the woman receives the needed support in labour and the puerperium which is normally the province of a midwife.

Midwifery care can be described as the planning and delivery of all midwifery care required for a client whoever her primary care provider might be. It would be possible therefore for a midwife acting as primary provider to provide all the care required for normal cases including the six week postnatal examination, but where general practitioners or obstetricians were the primary providers they would need to make arrangements for their clients to receive midwifery care. This raises the possibility of varying patterns of care in which the autonomy of the midwife over normal care is recognized. For example, women with obstetric problems require the oversight of an obstetrician at first, but are transferred to the care of midwives once a healthy outcome has been achieved.

Changing the status of midwives would have a number of effects upon other aspects of the service.

Antenatal care

Antenatal care would be provided by midwives in women's homes, in community- or hospital-based clinics, where the midwife would function as a practitioner rather than assisting the doctor. It was expected that this would dramatically reduce the pressure on hospital clinics, releasing medical time for the care of complicated cases, and thus improve the service for all clients.

Intrapartum and postnatal care

Midwives working as primary providers in delivery suites and postnatal wards would reduce the workload of junior doctors and improve the continuity of care for women. In many hospitals, although midwives conduct the labour, delivery and postnatal care of women, hospital routines require that junior doctors 'discharge' the women to their homes. This is not only inappropriate, but also it causes inconvenience to women who must 'wait to be discharged'. It may lead to problems in postnatal care when doctors have not been aware of the full needs of the woman. It has also been shown to increase hospital costs by inappropriate admission or retention of women in antenatal wards. Outcome evaluation (Ball, 1992) has shown that 25% or more of all admissions to delivery suites were 'false alarms', and that many women were kept in overnight or over a weekend by junior doctors who were unwilling to discharge them home, even though they were healthy and did not require any treatment.

Changes in the role of junior doctor

It was for these reasons that the proposals recommended that junior doctors should cease to have any responsibility in the care of normal pregnancies, but instead work under the direction of primary midwives and obstetric registrars, thereby gaining experience and skills in obstetrics. Midwives would refer directly to the obstetric registrar or consultant when the need arose.

Freeing midwives from wards and departments

Much of the work currently undertaken by midwives is concerned with the running of wards and departments. In the past, some types of work such as answering telephones, chaperoning duties, have been done by midwives mainly because there was no other type of staff available. The increasing use of health care assistants within the NHS is designed to release highly skilled staff from these duties. The introduction of health care assistants should be seen as a golden opportunity to free midwives to become increasingly client- rather than ward-centred.

In antenatal clinics health care assistants would take over chaperoning and reception duties, supporting doctors and midwives, dealing with medical records, laboratory reports, telephone calls, etc.

In delivery suites health care assistants on each shift would provide receptionist and domestic help, acting as first contact for telephone enquiries, so freeing midwives to concentrate on the care of mothers in labour.

In hospital wards health care assistants would provide a caring ambience, providing family type support to mothers and babies, while midwives provided the daily skilled attention in healthy low risk pregnancies. In some situations health care assistants could provide hotel type care to healthy women and babies between delivery and early transfer home to the care of the primary midwife. In wards caring for high risk pregnancies or ill women or babies health care assistants would work as support to the midwives.

Changes in the organization of midwifery care

Changing the status of midwives alone would not bring about the needed improvements in maternity care. It would be crucial to ensure that:

- Primary providers were not overloaded with work;
- Intrapartum care for all women was maintained at a high standard;
- Some means of co-ordinating and sharing care while not relinquishing the primary provider principle, should be found.

It was envisaged that midwives carrying their own caseload and providing services to their clients wherever needed (home, hospital or community services) would best fulfil the role of the primary provider. However, not all midwives would work in this way. There would be a need for other midwives, working alongside their group practice and medical colleagues as support or specialist midwives, providing the midwifery care and specialist skills for clients with complicated pregnancies and labours, and to ill neonates. To enable this to happen there was a need to end the current anomalies in the concepts surrounding the work of hospital- and community-based midwives. Instead it was recommended that midwives should work in group practices or hospital-based teams.

Group practice principles

Primary midwives would work in partnerships, group practices or teams, providing a 24 hour service to clients wherever needed. They would not be attached to specific wards or rotas within the hospital even though they would be likely to spend a good deal of time with their clients in the hospital setting. Instead of working to a $37^1/_2$ hour week, their workload would be controlled by their caseload size, and they would work on the basis of flexible working over the year.

Recommendations on caseload sizes

It was recommended that each group practice should consist of six midwives, taking joint responsibility for 200 cases per annum as primary providers, and also providing care to 85 women transferred for postnatal care by obstetricians and/or general practitioners. Within this group practice each full-time midwife would have primary responsibility for 30–40 women, with part-time staff taking a proportionately small caseload. The rationale for this size of caseload is shown in Fig. 5.2 and the total number of cases is reflected in the available hours per annum. This approach allows for flexibility of work required by the care of clients, whilst remaining within the recommended hours for whole-time equivalent staff. Basing the caseload on annual working hours is also helpful where job sharing takes place, or where part-time midwives form part of the group practice.

Principles of caseload and group practice management

- Within the total caseload of 200 cases, each midwife would be the primary provider and named midwife for 30–40 women per annum.
- Group practices would mainly be employed by provider units, but

We recommend a group of 6 midwives (4 primary and 2 associate) caring for 200 low risk cases per annum, and providing postnatal care for women for whom obstetricians were primary providers, on the basis of:

Primary	**time needed (in hours)**
Ante-natal care	
(as recommended by Hall, Mackintyre & Porter, 1985)	
Booking visit	1.5
9 further visits	7.00
Labour care	
Delivery	16
Post-delivery visit	1.0
Postnatal care	
2 visits on 2nd/3rd day	3.0
6 visits up to 9th day	3.5
4 further as needed	3.0
6 week visit	1.0
Total; direct care	36.0

To direct care time add 20% for administration, teaching and travel

   = 37.5 × 1.2
   = 45 hours

One WTE midwife works 37.5 hours per week × 45 weeks per annum

   = 1687.5 total hours per year which at 45 hours per case
   = 38 cases per annum

Also add 85 postnatal cases needing 10 hours of midwife time per case

   = 850 midwife hours per annum

Total caseload

   = 200 cases × 45 hours
   = 9000 hours + 850 postnatal hours
   = 9850 hours per annum

Number of midwives needed

   = 9850/1687.5 WTE midwife hours
   = 5.84 WTE midwives

Fig. 5.2 Caseload plans and costs of group practice. (Reproduced from Ball, *et al.*, 1992 with permission from the Nuffield Institute for Health, University of Leeds.)

they could also be self-employed or working in partnership with general practitioners.

- Each group practice would be required to have clear referral systems and protocols within which all primary and associate midwives would work.
- Each group practice would conduct regular peer reviews, establish clear audit systems, demonstrate effective, research-based practice and good care outcomes. Their group outcomes would be published.
- In each group practice a leader midwife would take part in policy-making for maternity services as a whole, participating in liaison committees with their medical and midwifery colleagues.

Controlling workloads and co-ordinating care

It will be important to be realistic in planning the work of caseload-based and specialist or support midwives. Work with midwifery managers in planning for the new type of service has revealed the danger of unrealistic expectations which could jeopardize the achievement of midwifery-centred and unified care. In particular, it will be essential to ensure that a high level of expertise is available at all times in delivery suites, and that caseload-based midwives are not overloaded with unrealistic workloads (Ball & Washbrook, 1993).

If one considers that 60–70% of all women fulfil low risk criteria, then in a unit providing care for 4000 births a year, based on an estimate of 65%, low risk cases would amount to 2600 per annum, and high risk cases (35%) would amount to 1400 per annum. If there were ten group practices (60 midwives), at 200 cases per annum per group, then they would be the primary providers for 2000 cases. This means that a further 600 low risk cases would need midwifery care in addition to the 1400 high risk cases booked by the obstetrician. Part of the answer might be to create more teams, but this would still leave the high risk women who would need specialist midwifery skills especially in intrapartum care. In the example given above, ten group practices would care for 2000 cases or 50% of all births.

Each group practice also provides postnatal care to 85 women per annum. In our example of 4000 cases per annum, therefore, group practices would provide all the care for 2000 women and the postnatal care for a further 850 women. This means postnatal care would still be needed for another 1150 women.

It can be seen that there is a clear need for specialist and support midwives to provide midwifery care for these cases, together with a pool of expertise in intrapartum care.

In the example given above, ten group practices would care for 2000 cases or 50% of all births. However, work undertaken in helping mid-wifery managers plan for the resources needed to implement the changes, suggests that group practice midwives would initially care for 30–40% of all women, and the Cumberlege Report (1993) recommends a target figure of 30% of all women having the midwife as the lead professional to be achieved over the next five years.

Specialist and support midwives

Specialist midwives would have particular expertise in intrapartum care, and in co-ordinating care of women between the different professionals during their stay in hospital. In addition to providing expertise in intrapartum care, e.g. oversight of epidurals, intensive care to complicated labours, teaching of student and intern midwives and junior doctors, they would provide a pool of expert advice to colleagues and act as co-ordinators of care. In this they would practise as primary providers of midwifery care, in liaison with their medical colleagues. Support midwives would work in hospital or community services, providing care to women in the absence of their primary provider midwives, e.g. night duty in hospital, overseeing care of women in wards. In addition other midwives will be needed to provide the community-based care for those women booked for obstetrician care as well as those low risk women who could not be accommodated within caseload work.

In all these situations there is potential for other team work based in either hospital or community, or linked to group practices.

Primary and associate midwives

'The basic principle underlying maternity care should be that a woman gets to know one midwife as "her midwife" and be assured that the bulk of her care will be carried out by her midwife' (Ball, *et al.*, 1992). The same principle is enshrined in the concept of the 'named midwife' (*Patient's Charter*, DoH, 1991). However, no single person can be on duty at all times and there would be need to provide a system of primary and associate midwives working in liaison to provide the co-ordinated care which Currell (1990) describes as 'unity' of care.

Within each service primary midwives would act as the named midwife and primary provider. Primary midwives would have the responsibility for planning and leading the care throughout pregnancy, labour and the puerperium. When the primary midwife was off duty or on leave, the care of the client would pass to the associate midwife. Associate midwives should not be seen as secondary midwives, they would maintain their practitioner status, and provide a major function in the co-ordinated care of mothers. There are many times in a midwife's career when she would prefer to work as an associate midwife. Those with teaching or management responsibilities could maintain their clinical skills as associate midwives as could midwives who might wish to work part-time to meet family responsibilities. Others might prefer to lay down the burden of primary provider responsibilities towards the end of their careers.

Changing career paths for midwives

Working within the framework outlined in the strategy would alter the present perceptions of care management and career patterns. Midwives would now work more fully as practitioners, being accountable for their own cases. The medical model of wards/departments run by Sisters in charge and staff midwives perpetuated a hierarchical structure which allocated decision making to the person with highest status or full time work. One only has to look at how ward rotas are written with the Sister and full-time staff listed first, and part-time staff lower, to see how this attitude is reinforced. This is not only unfair to experienced midwives working part-time or returning to practice after bringing up a family, it is also not efficient in making the best use of available skills. The unfairness and inappropriateness of this system was exposed when the grading system was introduced. Not only were there grades allocated which reflected the hierarchical status rather than the professional work undertaken, but there were also numerous anomalies between hospital- and community-based staff, and between different sets of community midwives. Some carried a caseload which included home or domino deliveries, others never delivered a baby but provided antenatal and postnatal care only.

Career paths

In order to address this issue and provide a pattern of career developments which would match the new status of midwives and their relationship with medical colleagues, a new pattern of career progression was proposed. This was designed to enable midwives to work in different patterns at different times without reducing the status or value of the experienced midwife.

Education

It was recommended that pre-registration training to diploma or degree level should become the norm for entry to the profession. Any continuing post-registration course for trained nurses should also be at diploma or degree level.

Stages of career development

It was proposed that, after qualifying, all midwives should enter the service via a six-month full-time or longer part-time *probationer* or *internship* system. At the end of this period midwives would move to *practitioner* status irrespective of part-time or full-time work. The status, function and grade would apply whether the midwife did most of her work in the hospital or community setting.

Practitioners would work as either primary or associate midwives in different settings. Consequently there should be an end to status titles such as Sister or staff midwife. The majority of midwives would work within the practitioner role.

The third level of midwifery practice would be that of the *expert* or *professional midwife*. This midwife might lead the work of several group practices, provide specialist midwifery skills, manage a total midwifery service or provide professional leadership via a research and/ or academic appointment. Such midwives would also undertake the role

Title	Equates to	Grade	Function role
Expert Midwife Practitioner/Professor	Consultant	Managerial/ clinical	Heads; several teams/ groups Specialist; CDU, neonatal services, directs services, etc.
		Grade begins at H or I	Professional support/ leadership; Research; Supervisor of midwives
Clinical leader 50% clinical + 50% teaching or 50% research	Registrar	G+	Heads; group practice, hospital department, some supervision duties.
Practitioner	Senior House Officer	F–G	Manages client caseload. Works as primary or associate midwife. Acts as resource for intern midwife/junior doctor, mentor for students.
Salary scales begin at F Intern midwife	House Officer	E	Newly qualified midwife, first 6 months

Fig. 5.3 Career progression, relationships and salary criteria. (Reproduced from Ball, *et al.*, 1992 with permission from the Nuffield Institute for Health Services Studies, University of Leeds.)

of supervisor of midwives and form the policy making/management body with their medical and manager colleagues.

Professional development criteria

It was recommended that all midwives holding primary provider or primary midwife posts undertake a fixed minimum number of deliveries per annum. Progression to the higher levels of expert midwife would be associated with undertaking research, or demonstrating increased clinical skills just as doctors do. The different levels of practice are shown in Fig. 5.3 above.

Pipe-dream or possibility?

At the time of publishing the strategy outlined in this chapter, there was considerable concern that the recommendations of the Winterton Report (1992) should be realized. Since that time there have been considerable amounts of activity which leads one to believe that midwives will at last be able to resume and extend their traditional practitioner role. The NHS Management Executive (NHSME) made the provision of midwifery beds one of the management objectives for 1993, and conducted a survey of midwifery and general practitioner-led units (NHSME, 1993). Several Regional and local health authorities and maternity units have set up consensus conferences and pilot group practice systems. Finally the Cumberlege Report (1993) has supported the proposals and set targets for their achievement over five years. This degree of activity and commitment to change is almost unprecedented within the health services of the United Kingdom. Now the realization of this dream lies in the hands of midwives at all levels.

Part 2
Creating Change

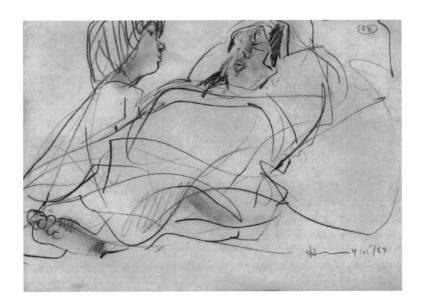

Chapter 6
Transforming the Organization

The nature of transformative change

What transformative change means

When people are transformed we say that they are different: they find new meaning in their lives, and often look and act differently. The same is true of the transformed organization. Organizational transformation requires a review of purpose, and in meeting this newly defined purpose people working within the organization find new ways of doing things. Transformation of an organization requires fundamental change at every level, of relationships between people, of employment practices, often of the structure of the organization.

In Britain, and in many other parts of the world, there is a call to transform the maternity services. This call is coming from the public, consumer groups, professionals and professional organizations, governments and those who control the funding of health care. There is a movement away from the medically dominated view of birth, toward giving women and their families control and choices in where their babies are to be born, who is to attend them, and their treatment. Women and professionals are also reviewing the advantages and disadvantages of particular forms of care, and are questioning much of the theoretical and scientific basis of obstetrical and midwifery care.

Earlier chapters bring out particular aspects of the transformed maternity services. The need for sensitive and personal care, the need for a trusting relationship between the woman and her caregivers, the need for a more thoughtful and scholarly approach to care, and of the utmost importance the need to recognize the nature of birth and its significance to individuals and families and the community. This chapter looks at the work of transforming the organization. It starts at the imaginative and creative beginnings, and goes on to the concrete nitty gritty work of making the change happen, of enabling people within the organization to live their vision in practice.

This chapter is written by four of us working in senior leadership positions in an organization which has created such a transformation.

We represent executive, professional, academic and business management roles; this representation is intentional, because transformation of an organization requires work in all corners and at all levels. The change will require adequate infrastructures, support and encouragement. Review and change of policy and practice will require close collaboration between many different people, and many sections of the organization.

Knowing your purpose and values

Most of us depend on familiar routines to live our lives and to guide our work. We have familiar roles, we know many of the people we work with, we perform tasks in a certain way following a particular pattern. Organizations work in the same way. People have particular roles, particular styles of communication. We tend to follow routines, perform tasks, and we have some sense of what is expected of us. Routines are necessary to help us live our everyday lives and do a job of work. But sometimes these routines become so mechanical, so thoughtless, that we remain busy without truly accomplishing what we should be doing.

Think of the average British maternity service. If you were to take a snapshot picture on any particular day you would see the following. Women who are pregnant see a number of different people, the average seems to be between 30–40. On discovering she is pregnant the women may register with her general practitioner, see the community midwives and go up to the hospital for antenatal checks. In hospital she may labour through several shifts of midwives and stay on the postnatal wards. Back home she is seen by community midwives and general practitioners once again. The woman proceeds through the service in the hands of a multitude of strangers. It seems almost self evident that this fragmented care should create problems. Firstly, although in Britain most women have a consultant in charge of their care, the woman may not even meet her consultant. Importantly, there is no one person in charge of her care. This means that there is no one person that she might contact with questions and concerns, who ensures that test results are back and acted on and that she knows the results. Furthermore, there is no one person to make continuous clinical judgements and decisions. But at the centre of the concern about lack of continuity is that there is no one person that the woman might form a relationship with, who she can know and trust, and who becomes her friend in the system.

These systems of care, apparently sensible and efficient, have operated for over 20 years in Britain. Routines which seemed productive went unchallenged. The ethos seemed well-intentioned. People knew what they were doing, how they should behave, who they should speak to, and the tasks they should be performing. Moreover the continuing improvement in perinatal survival made us feel that we were doing the right things, and doing them well. Then, suddenly it seemed, a clear sense of discontent arose. Women and their families, consumer groups and the public were saying that they were not content with the maternity services. This discontent seemed paradoxical given the apparently increased safety of birth (Winterton Report, 1992; Cumberlege Report, 1993). A pervasive sense of discontent amongst midwives has also been well documented over many years (Robinson, 1983). There has been a growing sense that professionals and the maternity services could be doing more for women, could be using their skills more appropriately. Accompanied as it has been by fundamental questions about the shaky scientific foundations of obstetrical and midwifery practice (Chalmers, *et al.*, 1989; Tew, 1990; Cumberlege Report, 1993), the questioning of the way our maternity services operate has pulled apart every aspect of care.

What has happened is that organizations have run in routine ways, being dominated by rules and routines: 'the rule of the rules', without examination or real review. Given that the hospital became the focus for the maternity services on such shaky evidence over 30 years ago, and that the organization may have been quite improperly skewed to an acute care model, we have veered far away from meeting the real purpose of our work. If an organization is a business relying on the selling of goods and services to the public, we soon know when we are selling or doing the wrong things, because people stop buying from us. It is not so clear in a public service, because in Britain anyway, the consumer is not always the person who is buying the service. It is because of this that organizations which serve the public need to review their purpose regularly or in reaction to indicators that all is not well.

This debate about purpose within the maternity services is vigorous both in Britain and many other parts of the world. So what is the purpose of our work? Many themes are emerging:

- The need to recognize that birth is a normal life event and is not a medical emergency.
- The need to put women to the centre of care and the organization so that they and their families have control and choice in where and how their babies are to be born.
- The need to support people in their emotional and social development as they become parents as well as providing physical care.

Our purpose therefore is not only to provide short term safety, but to be aware of the long term effects and potential benefits of our care.

The sense of purpose of an organization is closely intertwined with its values. If our purpose is to support families in choosing where and how their babies are to be born, and to support them in a healthy and happy start to parenting, these purposes are informed by particular values and will also lead, in a circular way, to different things being of value within the organization. It is strange how quickly we pick up the underlying values of an organization; these values can never really be hidden. If a maternity service, and the people working within it, really value giving women choices about place of birth, for example, you will find that staff will go to great lengths to support women in having a home birth or care in a community hospital. If organizations and the people working within them really value learning you will find lots of questioning and courses and books and videos and people sharing ideas.

If we recognize that giving birth is one of the most intimate and influential events of our life, and that parents need support in their transition to parenthood as well as physical care, you will find that the organization will value all sorts of human support in addition to the few medical procedures which are necessary around the time of birth. You will see evidence of these values in many different ways. You will see staff who are sensitive and skilled at communications, you will see professionals able to work in relationship with women and their families, treating them as the individuals they are and respecting their individual needs and wants. You will see rules and routines which work in the interests of families rather than the staff.

Changing the culture

We sense particular values and beliefs in the culture of the organization, as we might sense a different culture when we travel or go on holiday, in different parts of the world or even different parts of a country. For example, we might pick up quickly whether spontaneity or creativity is valued, or if children are valued, or if freedom of expression is valued. This change of culture is an important part of organizational change, and can be achieved intentionally, although not always easily. This awareness of the culture of an organization, and the effect it will have on staff and on care provided, is important. Peters & Waterman (1982) describe the importance of this culture as an expression of centrally held values, and describe how the wide adoption of particular values may replace the need for rules and regulations and complex procedures.

Let us give you an example. One of us visited a maternity service which valued 'woman-centred care'. This value pervaded everything, from the way women were asked in a matter of fact way where they would like their babies to be born to the involvement of women in policy and strategy for the service. It came through in the way women themselves talked about the service, in their sense of control, of happiness about the birth of their babies. The values were clear to the midwives too, who valued their role in the community. When a midwife was asked at the last minute to help a woman have a home birth, she could undertake that and call on colleagues to help. In contrast, where a service does not value a woman's right to have her baby where she chooses you will find inadequate systems to support the choice, and even when individual practitioners are willing to give women choices they might find they are unable to do so, or are unsupported if they do provide choices to the women they care for.

At a leadership level the culture is changed by showing what is of value to the organization in many ways. Value is demonstrated through what we spend our money on, the criteria which form performance reviews, the kind of behaviour which is praised and rewarded, the things we spend our time on. Similarly, at an individual level, values are expressed in our behaviour, attitudes, and what we spend our time on. For example, if a midwife in clinical practice values playing her full part in the service, and using all her skills and abilities, she will try to ensure she undertakes a number of deliveries, and does not just spend her time in postnatal visiting. But in order for her to do this, both she and the leaders of the service she practises in need the will to help her practise fully. There needs to be a general agreement that the full use of the midwife's skills is of value and importance.

Changing the structure

Transformation of an organization requires fundamental change at all levels of the organization (Beckhard, 1992). In the maternity services this may require that we radically change the way that midwives practise, so that rather than being allocated to wards and departments or the community, they carry a caseload.

Midwives in many parts of the world, particularly Britain, have been concerned over recent years to find the best structures, or patterns of practice, which would allow continuity of carer, and enable them to utilize all of their skills and abilities, in relation to individual women.

For over 13 years policy documents from government, professional associations and consumer groups have urged the need for more human approaches to care within the maternity services. All of these reports have called for greater continuity of care (see examples in Chapter 12). However, the concept has remained vague, and few people could think of how continuity could be enhanced given the restrictions of shift systems and the $37\frac{1}{2}$ week of midwives. It was the Know Your Midwife scheme started by Caroline Flint (Flint & Poulengeris, 1987) which showed a way that continuity could be improved, and got around the restrictions of the midwives' working week.

Other know your midwife schemes followed, and many team midwifery developments were initiated in many parts of the country. A few projects, for example the Kidlington Team in Oxford and the Riverside London teams, were set up on very similar lines to the Know Your

Midwife Scheme. In other words these were small teams, which integrated hospital and community. These projects had as their centrepoint the aim of providing continuity of care, as opposed to other developments which aimed to provide midwifery-led care.

Within ten years of the report of the Know Your Midwife scheme, 40% of maternity services had introduced organizational change within their units. Some were more successful than others, some schemes had to be abandoned (Wraight, *et al.*, 1993). Many of these developments have remained as pilots, and it seemed that teams, like the earlier domino deliveries, were never to spread so that continuity and midwifery-led care could become available to all women in the service and to all women in the country. Like domino schemes, team midwifery seemed doomed to remain experimental, or even to fizzle out.

But greater continuity of carer, and organizations which support continuity, will now be a necessary development within the maternity services. The Winterton Report (1992) provides detail on what it is that women want from the maternity services. It took the ideas of continuity further than other reports, and focused on the need for women to be in control over their own bodies and the birth of their own babies. Unlike other earlier reports it did not express blind faith in technology. It condemned all of the professions for their territorialism and lack of evidence-based practice. What was very important about this report was that it recognized the social nature of pregnancy and birth and the early weeks of life, and the social consequences of the way we care for families around the time they give birth to their babies. Winterton has irrevocably altered the framework for practice and scholarship within the maternity services.

Winterton described the need, expressed as a recurring theme by consumer groups, women themselves, and by many professionals, for women and their families to have choice, continuity and control in their maternity care: the three Cs. The report also called for a restoration of pride in the profession of midwifery, while deploring the obvious territorialism between the professions. In addition, the need for women to be informed and for care to be based on strong evidence where it exists was emphasized. It suggested that the work contained in *Effective care in pregnancy and childbirth* (Chalmers, *et al.*, 1989) should become a foundation for clinical practice.

The Expert Maternity Group was set up to review policy for the maternity services in England, as part of the Government's response to Winterton. The Cumberlege Report, the report of the Group, was published in August 1993. After a short period of consultation all its recommendations were accepted by the Government. The letter from the Chief Nursing Officer, Department of Health, and the Director of Health Care for the National Health Service Management Executive, circulated to all commissioners and providers of health care in England requires that the recommendations and targets within the report be reached within five years. In many ways the Cumberlege Report reflects the ideals expressed in Winterton, but takes them further, giving concrete targets and indicators of success.

But importantly, for those who really want to transform the care we offer childbearing families, the Cumberlege Report evokes a whole new spirit of care. It is this spirit which will need to be reflected in the culture of practice and in the atmosphere of the renewed maternity services, which will be as important as structural changes, and which will breath life into a new way of seeing our care around the time of birth. This new spirit and the way we put that spirit into practice, will put women and their families at the centre of the organization, giving them control over one of the most crucial events of their lives. It will also ensure that our care encompasses the responsibility of knowing where evidence exists to support our practice, and acknowledging where there is uncertainty. This new spirit of care will help us to find ways of making the maternity service accessible and attractive to all users in the community.

The very specific indicators of success shown in Fig. 6.1 give some idea of the kind of structural change which will be required in the maternity services in England in order to attain them.

The Cumberlege Report recommends very small teams, group practices or domino deliveries. There is room for experimentation and

---

(1) All women should be entitled to carry their own case notes.
(2) Every woman should know one midwife who ensures continuity of her midwifery care – the named midwife.
(3) At least 30% of women should have the midwife as the lead professional.
(4) Every woman should know the lead professional who has a key role in the planning and provision of care.
(5) At least 75% of women should know the person who cares for them during their delivery.
(6) Midwives should have direct access to some beds in all maternity units.
(7) At least 30% of women delivered in a maternity unit should be admitted under the management of the midwife.
(8) The total number of antenatal visits for women with uncomplicated pregnancies should have been reviewed in the light of the available evidence and the RCOG guidelines.
(9) All front line ambulances should have a paramedic able to support the midwife who needs to transfer a woman to hospital in an emergency.
(10) All women should have access to information about the services available in their locality.

Fig. 6.1 Changing childbirth: indicators of success. (Reproduced from the Cumberlege Report, 1993 with permission.)

evaluation. In the Centre for Midwifery Practice at Queen Charlotte's and Hammersmith Maternity Service, we have implemented the following model of care, which we call one-to-one midwifery practice. This model is characterized by the following:

- Midwives working in partnerships within group practices of six midwives.
- Each midwife carries a caseload of 35–40 births a year.
- The named midwife ensures her partner gets to know her families so that on call can be covered.
- Women choose their lead clinician: midwife, general practitioner or obstetrician.
- If there are complications care is by an obstetrician.
- The midwife is named midwife for everyone in her caseload, so sometimes she is lead clinician, sometimes she provides midwifery support which includes, care in labour and for the birth of the baby

The term 'one-to-one' signifies two things. First, it recognizes the potential of a special relationship between woman and midwife. This relationship should enable sensitivity to the needs of the individual woman and her family. We aim to make this possible through the 'one-to-one' approach. Not all care will be provided by this one midwife, and she does not have to be constantly available, but she is still the anchor of good care and the friend in the system, and plans and provides much of the care herself.

The second thing that one-to-one care signifies is that there is one midwife who is responsible for ensuring a woman and her family receive all their care appropriately, and that that care is planned together with the woman.

This organization puts into practice many of the recommendations of the Cumberlege Report. It provides all women within the project with a named midwife, who follows them through the system, and who is directly available by mobile phone. If the named midwife is unavailable the midwife's partner takes the call. The approach also links care in hospital and community, and allows women to choose between midwife-led or doctor-led care.

There are several well-known patterns of practice, including team midwifery, domino deliveries, group practices, which have all supposedly been aimed at improving continuity of care. There are still some unanswered questions about these new patterns of practice. For example, what is the ideal number of midwives in a team or group to allow the woman to have a real relationship with her named midwife, and a genuine relationship with her accoucheur? How do we balance the needs of the woman with the needs of her attendants, and how much on call is it reasonable to expect a midwife or doctor to do? If the

team is too large it is less likely that the woman will know her accoucheur and communications become more time consuming and
complex. If the team is small then there is a greater on call requirement,
but communications are simpler, less time consuming, and calls while
on duty should be fewer. Some argue that a minimum of four midwives
is necessary because a smaller number means that the system is more
likely to fail, making the known midwife or midwives unavailable in a
crisis and leaving the woman disappointed. Domino deliveries in most
services were doomed to failure because it seemed nobody thought of
reorganizing the service to give back-up to midwives who were known
to the woman and it was a hit and miss approach to having the woman's
own midwife with her for labour and birth.

The chosen pattern of practice may vary according to the needs of
individual populations, the geography and size of the maternity service.
But there are some guiding principles to deciding on the pattern. The
first is that you should be clear what the purpose of the new pattern is. If
it is to provide a trusted and familiar face for each woman for care
throughout pregnancy and for times of anxiety or crisis and for labour
and birth, then small numbers are required for the woman's care group.
A maximum of six is recommended (Wraight, *et al.*, 1993), although
four or five may be better (Cumberlege Report, 1993). In our service we
are trying partnerships, with a named midwife for each woman, and the
midwife partner getting to know the woman too, so she can be available
when the named midwife is off call. These partners work within a group
practice, for support, caseload allocation and peer review. We shall be
carefully monitoring the number of times the woman gets her named
midwife, the partner or somebody unknown to her for the birth of the
baby. We shall also be monitoring the feelings of the midwives as they
take on these caseloads. Each midwife has a caseload of 35–40 births a
year, allocated according to expected dates of delivery to ensure each
midwife has clear breaks.

Our pattern of practice will allow women to choose who they wish
their lead practitioner to be. So some women will be receiving midwifery-led care. Thus we are bringing into play two aims, the provision
of a known and trusted professional for care, and the possibility of
midwifery-led care.

If continuity of carer is the main aim then hospital and community
care should be integrated, and midwives should be comfortable and
competent practising in each. The midwife should feel able to be with
the woman where and when wanted. In other words, we need to do
away with the barriers of ward and departmental allocation and strict
and inflexible shift systems. Finally, the midwife continues to be the
woman's named midwife even when there are complications (although
a specialist or 'consultant midwife' may be called upon to assist with care
and will work in collaboration with a doctor.

Deciding where you are going

Processes of clarification

We hope by now that it is clear that the kind of change we are talking about, the kind of change which will bring about transformation is fundamental in its nature, changing both structures and cultures within the service. This change, which relies on us being clear of our social purpose, may be difficult to achieve in a slow and incremental manner, because slow, incremental changes really only work in slow-moving, stable societies (Beckhard, 1992).

Fundamental change requires looking at all parts of the organization with a view to changing them all. This does not mean that the change should be ad hoc. Fundamental change requires that we are very clear where we are going and how we will get there. In other words the purpose and aim of the change should be clear, we should be clear of the principles we wish to put into practice, and we should examine what it is that we really value. Such change needs strategic direction and constant review to make sure you are not going off the tracks. It does mean working out steps and which order they should be taken in, which is not the same thing as sitting in the office doing detailed planning in isolation. It is much more a constant cycle of talking, thinking, watching, listening, trying out ideas, and profound discussion with both protagonists and antagonists. Of course there is a place for systematic planning, but planning should not be overdone: it is one part of a complex process.

Working groups, away days, missions and critical paths

At some point, values and abstract ideals or principles have to be put into practice. In other words, the day-to-day operation of the service should demonstrate such principles as 'woman-centred care, accessibility of the service, effective and efficient care' (Cumberlege Report, 1993). Much of the work of clarifying purpose and values and then seeing how they should be put into practice can be undertaken by working groups. These working groups should not consist only of senior managers, but should also have strong representation from the 'coal face', people who know what the everyday problems will be. Importantly, there should be strong consumer representation on these working groups. It goes without saying that it helps if a number of the people on the working group are also committed to overcoming the inevitable problems.

There are several techniques that can be used to develop principles into practice and these can help groups focus on translating thoughts into actions. By having a vision of the future of specific elements of the service you could use a SWOT (strengths, weaknesses, opportunities, threats) analysis. This consists of looking at the strengths and weaknesses of what is currently provided which tends to have an internal focus for the organization. From this comes a consideration of the opportunities the new ideas will bring, together with a view on the possible threats to the proposed service. This later undertaking has a more external focus to it, and it stimulates the development of strategies to maximize available opportunities and minimize threats.

Another model we have found useful is Lewin's driving analysis (Lewin, 1951). This technique recognizes that resistance to change is a natural phenomenon and therefore it is worth examining in detail where resistance is likely to occur to both highlight what is occurring and to indicate what could be done to bypass problems. The technique aims to focus on the forces, or individuals, for and against change. By describing these forces and assigning them different weights, it is possible to draw up a grid of areas, groups and individuals and to identify how much resistance is likely to be felt. The resulting grid enables you to develop a strategy for defeating or lessening individual strands of resistance.

Every so often the group needs to get away for clear spans of time to do some real talking and thinking away from the daily pressures of the organization. With an outside facilitator who will ask searching questions, seek clarification and challenge, one day away can be worth a week in time. David Marlow, the Chief Executive of the Hammersmith and Queen Charlotte's Special Health Authority, took the action group from the Centre for Midwifery Practice out for a day soon after its inception, helping us to defend ideas, explain and clarify what it was that we were trying to do. The result of the day's work was a short mission statement:

> 'to seek ways of promoting excellence in midwifery practice which provide an individual service to women and their families, respecting their rights, beliefs and values.'

The work and thinking that went into this statement laid the foundations for change, and made many subsequent decisions easier. There will always be difficult questions to answer, and genuine dilemmas, but they really are easier to resolve with some clarity of purpose and through knowing what is of value.

In addition to this 'visionary' work, some profound thinking needs to go on about the critical path for change. In other words, you will need to work out what is critical and at which point decisions need to be made and actions taken. Some people are good at putting these 'critical paths' on paper, but they are rarely left unchanged, and should be dynamic and flexible. Much of this is obvious. For example, you need to know how much money you will need and where it will come from, how many staff you will need and where they will come from, the kind of development they will need, the level of salaries they will be paid, and what their pattern of practice will be.

Policies, guidelines for referral and guidelines for practice also need to be worked out. One important aspect of this fundamental change, if it is being undertaken in one part of the organization at a time, will be to work out how the rest of the service will be kept running efficiently and without feeling too deprived by the innovation. All this work is complex, time consuming, and needs a number of people from different backgrounds to work on it. Finance staff, personnel or human resources departments, teachers, transport and security officers all play a crucial part in such a change. We found that these members of the team were often really enthusiastic about the ideas we were working out, and because they could see the end point, gave great commitment and really helped to move the project forward.

Consultation

Consultation can be a tricky business, but real and genuine consultation is essential. Where do you start? After a difficult meeting one evening when we were at a crucial stage in implementing one-to-one midwifery care, we decided that consultation was like one of those pin ball games, where you ping one pin then another, but sometimes you fail and you end up at the beginning again. Before starting on any organizational change there are certain groups you have to have on your side. But as soon as you start to talk to one group, rumours are flying and everyone knows or imagines what is happening. The key is to identify the stakeholders you have to convince before getting started so that you know you have some grass roots support. Although you can never expect everybody to want the change, it is important to stay sensitive to misunderstandings, worries, and even intentionally planted rumours. Consultation is as much art as science, requires a lot of attention, and sensitivity and sympathy for worries, while keeping the whole thing positive.

Consultation over changes in the maternity services, where both primary and secondary health care teams are involved are particularly complicated. We felt we were doing quite well with our consultation process, and seemed to be getting a lot of support for quite a complex and fundamental change. But our service affected a lot of general practices in our local catchment area. We had attempted to meet with these doctors for some time, to talk through our proposals, to no avail. Then at the eleventh hour the general practitioners seemed to realize the impact the change in service would have for them, and the whole development was almost stopped. It took a long time and quite sensitive negotiation to get some common basis of understanding and agreement on the principles and process of the change. In retrospect we should have pushed for face-to-face discussions with individual general practitioners at the beginning. But the process of consultation involves many stakeholders, and sometimes it is easier to think that non response is agreement, and to welcome escape from discussion about contentious issues.

There are two important points to make. The first is that the maternity service is a public service which has a powerful effect on the individuals and families it serves, so we must be clear when we undertake change that we should be working in the public interest. Close involvement of public representatives, consumer groups and a knowledge of the characteristics of local populations are essential. In Britain we are guided in this process by the purchasers of health care, whose job it is to know of general public needs, and to give specifications for the kind of service it wishes to buy.

A formal planned process of consultation is essential. Without it planning occurs in a vacuum and those you thought might be supportive are likely to change their minds at a critical point. It helps to have this process of consultation led from the executive level, with a lot of input from the human relations or personnel departments. This process of consultation consists of the circulation of discussion documents, of meetings, of one-to-one discussion, presentations and roadshows. The consultation occurs with consumers usually through consumer groups or perhaps through questionnaires. It also involves purchasers, local doctors, family health service authorities, and other providers and stakeholders in the service.

There will always be people who will oppose change – this is part of our nature as human beings – but it is often from the resisters of change that we learn where the real problems of the change will be and we are actually helped in working things out by honest discussion.

At some point in the consultation process agreement is reached about the general aims and guiding principles of the change. Then, concerns and objections can be taken into account, but within some parameters. Early discussion documents might be filled in and refined once the process of consultation is well underway, taking into account the results of discussions which have been part of the consultation process. Our preliminary consultation document for one to one care became the final consultation document, and then formed the business plan which went to the Executive Board and the Special Health Authority for final approval.

Be prepared to defend and discuss your ideas. This can be difficult because those who care enough to undertake and lead fundamental change put out to public scrutiny by peers, senior staff, colleagues, friends and foes, their most cherished convictions. When these convictions are questioned and opposed it can feel as if you are being attacked personally. Eventually, with experience and a thicker skin it becomes easier to defend and persuade without feeling personally attacked, and often people are (and have to be) won over. One thing to remember is that it is not the people who will argue with you face-to-face who will stop a change from happening, it is those who avoid you like the plague, who never come to meetings, and who will, at the eleventh hour, say they knew nothing about the change and that they were never consulted. Just in case, always keep good records of the circulation of documents, dates of meetings and so on.

Putting change into practice

Developing a business plan

Within the reformed NHS, proposed developments should be written up in much the same way as a commercial development should be, with a business plan. Study of previous NHS examples is useful when embarking on the production of a business plan, but hints from the commercial world can also be helpful (Scholes & Kleman, 1977; West, 1988; Barrow & Barrow, 1988).

The service plan lays out the mission or purpose and aims of the new organization. It describes how the aims will be translated into objectives to be achieved. It must show how the proposed development has grown from an examination of what services are required by the population for which it is to be provided, as elucidated nationally through governmental initiatives such as the Cumberlege Report (1993) and the 1992 White Paper entitled 'The Health of The Nation' or, more locally, purchasers' specifications. Evidence of market research, both local and national, helps to build up the case for your project. Do search the literature and keep an eye on what your competitor providers are offering: there is little point in claiming an innovative approach if you are merely duplicating the efforts of others.

The business plan also is the document in which the day-to-day operation of the service is described. A key section will be that detailing the resources required: staff, premises, capital equipment, consumables and any other running costs. Also essential will be the proposed quantity and quality of service these resources will buy. The minimum standard will be that of the status quo, but purchasers will be seeking to see tangible benefits in terms of increased volume of service, or improved quality. Standards for quality are therefore required to be set, and the business plan should include how these will be monitored. Take care therefore to ensure standards are set which can actually be measured, such as improving continuity of care by reducing the number of professionals in contact with a woman during her maternity care. Do ensure also that the measurement of these standards does not become so costly or time-consuming as to defeat the object!

It helps if the business plan is brief and to the point, especially because most of us working in public services cannot cope with the paperwork we are faced with. It also helps if it is well presented and eye catching. Making the plan brief can be difficult if you are one of the people who has gathered ideas, and worked with the complexity of the proposed change, because the complexity has to be simplified. A good critical reading by a trusted and honest colleague before the business plan is submitted is essential.

Costing

In developing one-to-one care for almost a quarter of the population we serve we were shifting resources from different parts of the organization to another. To put it crudely we were deciding to spend money on different things. Removal of midwives to the demonstration project from other parts of the service, different grades, mobile telephones, transport and equipment all had to be funded from within the existing money. Thus accountants and financial directors need to be involved in such a development from the beginning to work out costs, and to help identify where resources might be released. In our case money was shifted by the closure of some beds, by predicting a shorter length of stay for those women being cared for within the Centre for Midwifery Practice. We felt this was justified because if women feel supported they are likely to be willing to go home early, sometimes as early as a few hours after the birth of the baby, and to identify when they need help. The skill mix of ward, out patients department, and delivery suite, was also changed to reflect the shift of work to the community and community based midwives, and the effect of the presence of Centre for Midwifery Practice midwives. Staffing savings were also identified in additional time for medical and clerical staff to spend on other tasks which would have required an increase in staff without the project. Bed closures also meant savings on cleaning, catering and other support service overheads. The empty bed space was not wasted but was utilized to provide hotel beds for mothers with babies in the neonatal unit and a day area for antenatal patients requiring monitoring or minor procedures. Neither of these services could be provided adequately previously due to the usual pressures on space.

This working out all has to be done while keeping key people in the organization informed and involved. This is possibly one of the most complicated and crucial areas when undertaking change. And in most health services all over the world it is unlikely that you will get started if the development will cost too much. Beware, because often there is a mistaken feeling that new developments will be too costly, but when they are worked out they might actually cost the same or less than the traditional service. With costs do not make assumptions, get a professional who knows finances to help work them out. You will need to differentiate between fixed and variable costs so you examine ways of funding, or the difference varying the size of the project makes.

There is always somebody who buys and somebody who provides the maternity service. In independent midwifery practice the relationship is direct. The woman buys the services of a midwife or perhaps a group of midwives. Before the reforms of the NHS in Britain the maternity services were funded by the unit that they were in, and that money came down from regional to district level. Now, there is a clearer split between the commissioners of health care, that is the purchasers, and the providers. This has led to a more formal approach to contracting between the two elements, and as the roles are becoming more developed specifications for services are becoming more sophisticated.

Some awareness of this process is important for several reasons. Firstly, this gives some guidance to the kind of change which will be acceptable. Secondly it makes clear that purchasers should be an important and central part of any consultation. Purchasers are important allies, particularly given their responsibility for the local community's overall health needs, and the more progressive organizations will be open to good ideas about how change in the maternity services might be brought about.

Leading the way

Sharing the vision, keeping the vision, and living the vision

In the successful organizations surveyed by Peters & Waterman (1982) the direction, and the work of the organization was kept together and inspired by a shared vision, a commitment to the values of the organization. Much of the work of successful leadership is the ability to create or encourage a clear vision of where change should and will lead. But describing and sharing the vision is one thing, putting it into practice is another. This requires a mixture of imagination, of being in tune with the times, of having worked out what living the vision in reality will mean. After that it requires tireless determination and political skill. But it also requires that the vision, the picture of what the service will be like, is accepted, shared and put into practice by the majority of people working in the organization. This in itself requires a complex process of change in structures, in attitudes, in working relationships, and sometimes in buildings. If, for example, we wish to create a service which is woman-centred we need receptionists who will look up and smile when a woman approaches a desk, and who know that they should put the needs of an anxious woman above the need of an irate professional. We also need bigger and bolder steps. If, for example, a woman wishes a midwife rather than a doctor to lead her care we need to help the midwife and doctor work out different ways of working together, to help the midwife practise effectively. It is far easier to slip back into old ways of working once the chips are down than to keep the vision in mind and in practice.

Working in partnership

For many years midwives have worked in hierarchical, and controlling relationships. This has meant that change has been directed from the top, through the chain of command, leaving those at the woman's side little room even for clinical decision-making. The changes which have been proposed for the maternity services from a number of sources require that we enable those midwives who are in clinical practice to work with women, making decisions about care together with the women themselves. It calls for greater autonomy for the midwife, but at the same time a greater personal and professional accountability.

In this situation midwifery leadership needs to become enabling, and senior midwives need to learn to work in partnership with midwife clinicians. Perhaps one of the greatest strides will be when midwifery leaders continue to practise, just as doctors in leadership positions do, and do not have to adopt the clip board to climb the professional ladder. But this is a two way process, for the giving up of the controlling approach to management will require that all midwives adopt a self-determining attitude to practice, professional development, time and resource management, and in the creation of change.

Steering and enabling

Proposing this flat management structure is not the same as saying that all staff have the same function within the organization, because there are different functions to be performed. One of the most important parts for the leader of any organization to play is keeping an overview, to keep the service responsive to public and political demands, and to keep the central values and purpose of the organization alive and in practice. This allows a balancing between the seemingly opposed functions of enabling and supporting, while steering or guiding the direction of the organization.

Letting go of control

The world we live in is complex and fast changing. The reforms we are talking about require a complex matrix of change. No one person can know everything that is going on or remain in charge of everything. The ability to let go of control is one of the greatest skills of a leader. This requires careful selection of staff, staff who have the personal, intellectual and political skills to put complex changes into operation. This letting go happens at every level. In Chapter 11 two midwives who have been clinical leaders in setting up and running midwifery practices describe their role. It is through these roles that the vision becomes reality. They must be undertaken by people who work at every level of the organization, but who are mainly concerned with putting ideas into operation in the place of practice, working out resources and systems and support. But these people too must learn to give up control, helping midwives in practice to accept that they manage their own caseload, their own practice, their own time and equipment. We are pushing power and the authority for making decisions down to the midwife clinicians who work with the woman, on the assumption that this power will be used to empower the woman and her family. At every level this requires trust and helping others acquire the skills for their increased responsibility, their autonomy and accountability.

Politics and public relations

Conflicts and tensions

Politics with a small 'p' enter every area of our lives. They are especially prominent for anyone taking forward change at the level we are discussing. Even when people agree on a goal, they may see a different way of reaching it. And not everyone will have the same goal in mind. It is the politics of different people approaching things in different ways, or reaching for different goals which create the politics of change. Such politics create conflict and tension. But it is important to realize that such tension is an inevitable part of change, and may be a continuing and inevitable part of every dynamic organization. Any midwife, whether she is acting as advocate for a woman she is caring for in delivery suite, or setting up group practices, has to have political skills. These skills involve an awareness of what is going on in the world outside and in the wider organization, of knowing what is important to fight for, and what to leave alone, and when to fight for major issues. Skills of communication (including listening), of persuasion and debate are important. Importantly they also involve an ability for self protection, and for keeping one's own integrity.

Importance of support from above and below

The kind of change we are describing includes changes in power relationships, in allocation of resources, and in the structure of the organization. It is change with major implications and is very risky.

Change makes everyone nervous, not only those opposed to it but also those who want it. It is like being excited about moving to a new and better house but knowing you will miss your neighbours or the walk down the block or the view from the kitchen window. You want to change, but sometimes wonder if you should. Firstly anxieties about the change have to be aired honestly and not discounted. This helps them to be dealt with adequately.

Because change makes people nervous it requires real commitment from those at the top of the organization, the chairman and executives and directors. At the same time change requires grass roots support. Kanter (1984) provides many examples of how the most promising of changes cannot survive without the real will of those who lead the organization, and also how the most clearly thought out and imaginative changes cannot be put into practice without the support of a critical mass at the grass roots level.

We have talked about the need to work in the public interest, to know what it is that women and their families want from us when they have their babies. We need to be sensitive to their individual dreams, fears and wishes. We need to be able to respond to the altered meanings of birth in a fast changing society. We work in service to the public, and so our change should take us to the point where our maternity services are of the community they serve, responding to its needs. So the leaders of the maternity service, and the professionals who practice within it, are the servants of the public and the families they care for. When our change takes us to the point where this is recognized in practice we will have succeeded and our service will be truly transformed.

Chapter 7
Continuity of Carer in Context: What Matters to Women?

Introduction

In this chapter I would like to focus mainly on women's views and experiences of continuity of carer – that is women having the chance to get to know those who care for them during the childbearing period, and getting care from known care-givers at crucial times. This is a more specific and useful concept than the term 'continuity of care' which can include improved communication between care-givers, or individualized care (Murphy Black, 1992; Currell, 1990; Wraight, *et al.*, 1993). But continuity of carer is only one aspect of good personal care. Research about women's experiences of maternity care points to the need for care that is informative, accessible, respectful, supportive and competent. The chapter looks at the evidence from surveys and experimental studies about women's views and experiences of continuity of carer and then describes research about women's priorities for maternity care.

In preparing this chapter, the small number of relevant randomized controlled trials were identified from the Cochrane Pregnancy and Childbirth Database of Systematic Reviews. In addition many surveys and other non-experimental studies have been carried out and some important but unpublished studies will have been missed. In addition, studies may have been carried out where continuity of carer was not the main focus but was achieved as an important by-product, making it hard to be sure that all the relevant work has been found.

Evidence about women's experiences and views on continuity of carer

Some surveys have covered women's experiences of, and views on continuity of carer. Researchers have looked at different aspects of continuity. Some studies have asked whether the woman felt that she had got to know her care-givers, or whether she had already met the people caring for her at particular times. For example, in a study based in Cambridge, 24% of the 710 women from six different maternity units who filled in a postnatal questionnaire reported that they had previously

96

met at least one of the midwives who cared for them in labour (Green, *et al.*, 1988). In the Know Your Midwife scheme, just under half the women in the standard care group saw fewer than 8 care-givers in pregnancy, compared to nearly 80% of those in the know your midwife group (Flint, 1991).

A source of recent data on many aspects of women's experience of care is the pilot study carried out to test the Survey Manual, Women's Views of Maternity Care (produced by the Office of Population Censuses and Surveys (OPCS) (Mason, 1989). This showed that between 15% and 28% of women said that they had met any of the doctors and midwives who cared for them in labour (unpublished data).

Some studies have asked about a very minimal form of continuity of carer, for example, whether one midwife had been able to stay with a woman through the whole of her labour and delivery. It may seem very limited as an aim, but women's comments do show that it matters to them. In the Know Your Midwife report several women commented on this aspect of their care. One woman wrote:

> 'I found I was seen by too many midwives and doctors. When I went into labour I had one midwife, then it was staff changeover, then I had two different ones. I think this should be changed as you can't build up a relationship with someone when you have too many staff looking after you.'
>
> (Flint & Poulengeris, 1987)

In their trial, women in the know your midwife group saw fewer midwives in labour, on average, than women having standard care. And from the Cambridge study, 66% of women reported that at least one midwife was present from start to finish (Green, *et al.*, 1988).

Women who are classified as being at extra risk may particularly need continuity of carer. However, in a study of women who had had at least one previous low birthweight baby, Oakley (1991) found that those women who had had two or more low birthweight babies saw more care-givers in the course of their antenatal care than did those having low risk pregnancies.

The questions used to canvass women's feelings and opinions about continuity of carer are also quite varied. The OPCS pilot study questionnaire asked 'Would you like to have got to know them [the doctors and midwives who cared for you in labour] before going in?' Between 15% and 31% said yes definitely (unpublished data). In a survey carried out in several districts in one region, Melia *et al.* (1991) found that 46% of women replying to a postnatal questionnaire thought that it was very important to have the same team of midwives antenatally and post-natally. A further 31% thought that this was quite important.

Comments from mothers involved in the Know Your Midwife scheme

(Flint & Poulengeris, 1987) make it clear that improved continuity was really important for some women in the scheme. The scheme also appeared to lead to care that was informative, accessible and supportive. For example:

> 'I think that the Know Your Midwife scheme is best because you build up a friendly close relationship over the months and this I feel puts you at ease.'

> 'Lots of help and advice has been given and friendly faces are always around – it makes you feel special.'

> 'They seem to have more time for you, and tend to treat you as a person as well as a patient.'

> '... the scheme has been beneficial in terms of getting to know midwives and amount of time spent at clinics – long may it last.

Some survey research about women's views of care provides strong but indirect support for improved continuity of carer. I will mention two aspects of women's views – their preferences for locally provided care and their unhappiness about conflicting advice.

First, let us consider women's preference for locally provided care. Several researchers have compared women's opinions about antenatal care in hospital clinics to those about care provided locally by general practitioners and midwives. In a national sample survey of over 2000 women carried out in the late 1970s (O'Brien & Smith, 1981) striking differences emerged between the care provided in hospital and community settings.

Hospital clinics were more difficult to get to, and appointments took much longer. On average, women were more satisfied with care in the community and this can be partly explained by the fact that the community-based care was much more likely to have been provided by the same one or two people at each visit. Women in either setting who had care from the same one or two people at each visit were more likely to say that their medical and midwifery care was very good; that their treatment as a person was very good; that the staff were very good about explaining things; and that they felt able to discuss things.

In the pilot study carried out to test the OPCS Survey Manual mentioned above, questions about the personal content of care showed that local antenatal check-ups came out better on average than hospital check-ups. Far more women said that at most local check-ups there was 'someone who has got to know you and remembers you' (Garcia, 1989).

Turning now to the issue of conflicting advice: women's unhappiness about conflicting advice emerged in some of the early studies about maternity care (e.g. Morris, 1960, Oakley, 1979) and more recent work has given examples of the problems that it can cause for women in relation to, say, breastfeeding. Here is a comment written by a woman involved in a survey carried out by Josephine Green and her colleagues in Cambridge (Green, *et al.*, 1988):

'The staff treated me as though my brain had been removed, with regard to breastfeeding. I was told: 1) feed as long as you like, 2) 15 minutes one side then change for next feed, 3) 8 minutes each side, 4) 5 minutes each side, 5) not to feed more than once every 5 hours, 6) feed whenever you like. This "information" was all on the day of the birth and from different staff.'

The pilot study for the OPCS Survey Manual provides evidence that conflicting advice is experienced by a substantial number of women, at least in the postnatal period. In the questionnaire that was administered postnatally women were asked: 'In hospital, after the birth were you ever confused or worried because the different staff were giving you different advice?' In the four pilot districts, between a third and a half of women answered yes to this (Garcia, 1989).

Women's priorities for care

Just how important is continuity of carer to women, when compared with other aspects of care? Research about women's views of care has not generally been good at tackling the issue of the importance that women attach to various aspects of the care that they get.

For example, take an issue which quite often arises in conversations with women who have had a baby – being left alone by staff during labour. One could address this by asking women if they have been left alone at any time, or one could go a step further and ask, 'Were you ever left alone when it upset you to be left alone?'. This would get a bit closer to what women felt about it. In an interview (probably with a small number of women), the researcher could explore further and find out more about the times when a woman was left alone, and what was or was not upsetting. Another approach would be to ask women to put some sort of ranking on their feelings about different aspects of care. 'Not being left alone in labour' could be put alongside topics like 'being cared for by a midwife you know' and 'getting explanations of what is happening' and each could be ranked on a scale from essential to very undesirable. This provides extra information for service providers but takes a step away from women's actual experiences and towards more hypothetical choices.

One study carried out in a consultant maternity hospital (Drew *et al.*, 1989), asked women who had had a baby in the last few days to score

40 aspects of maternity care on a scale from essential to irrelevant. Midwives and obstetricians also used the scale to record their assessment of what was important to women. Only two items among the 40 referred to continuity of carer. These were: being attended by the same midwife during pregnancy, and being attended by the same doctor during pregnancy. These two were ranked by women (and care-givers) as of middling importance scoring respectively 21 and 23. At the top of the list came the baby being healthy, and two items about communication. These were: the doctors talking to you in a way you can understand, and having all your questions answered by staff. There is no item in this study that asks about having a known carer during labour.

From the Cambridge study of women's expectations and experiences of labour (Green *et al.*, 1988), some idea can also be gained of how important women thought it would be to have a known care-giver in labour. Women were asked a series of questions and Table 7.1 gives the

Table 7.1 Women's preferences for care in labour, assessed antenatally. (Source: Green, *et al.*, 1988.)

	Questionnaire	% Yes	Number
Question	Do you want a birth companion (husband/partner/ mother/friend) with you at all times throughout labour?	94	700/742
Answer	Yes, I want this very much, *plus* Yes, I would quite like this.		
Question	How important is it to you to be sure that you do not make a lot of noise during labour?	42	313/737
Answer	Very important, *plus* Quite important		
Question	Do you want to be looked after during labour by a midwife that you have already met?	62	457/737
Answer	Yes, I want this very much, *plus* Yes, I would quite like this		
Question	Do you want to have the same midwife with you throughout your labour and delivery?	87	640/737
Answer	Yes, I want this very much, *plus* Yes, I would quite like this		
Question	How important is it to you not to have lots of different people coming in and out of the room while you are in labour?	87	640/738
Answer	I definitely do not want (this), *plus* I would prefer not to have (this)		
Question	Do you want to be in control of what doctors and midwives do to you during your labour?	82	600/733
Answer	Yes, I want this very much, *plus* Yes, I would quite like this		

percentages of women answering 'yes'. Being attended in labour by a midwife they had already met did not rate as highly as some other items.

A recent national face-to-face interview study was carried out by MORI's Health Research Unit for the Expert Maternity Group (Rudat, *et al.*, 1993). Women were included in the survey if they had had a baby in the UK since 1 April 1989. In the MORI survey, women were asked, 'If you went through a pregnancy and birth again, what would matter most to you in terms of the care you were given?' The replies are given in Table 7.2

The question was an open one – there were no preset categories for women to choose from. Nineteen per cent mentioned some aspect of continuity of carer, and 13% wanted more information or explanation. The next two categories were about the need for caring and reassurance and scored 13% and 8% respectively.

Two other aspects of personal care were each mentioned by about 8% of women. Making sure that the baby is alright was mentioned spontaneously by only 7% of women, in contrast to the ranking it got in the previous study where it was one of the categories offered to mothers. Perhaps women took it for granted as one of the main features of care. So overall, continuity comes out from this study as being one of the most important things that women want from their maternity care.

In Ann Oakley's study of women who had had a low birthweight baby

Table 7.2 Women's preferences for care in labour, assessed postnatally. Base: all women (1005 women, national sample). (Source: Rudat, *et al.*, 1993.)

If you went through a pregnancy and birth again, what would matter most to you in terms of the care you were given? (Responses from 7% or more of women taking part.)

Answers	%	Number
Continuity/seeing same midwife or doctor	19	193
More information/explain what is involved	13	133
More caring/understanding/support	13	126
More reassurance	8	82
Listen to your views/treated as a person	8	84
More personal attention	6	85
More/regular checks/tests	7	72
Making sure baby was alright	7	69
None/no problems/satisfied	8	85
Don't know	7	66

Table 7.3   Preferences of women who had had a low birthweight baby. (Source: Oakley, 1991.)

Was there anything you felt you needed in the way of support or help during that time that you didn't have?

Answers	% Yes
More information from doctors	58
More continuity of care	42
More sympathetic medical care	37
Financial help	23
Help with housing	23

(1991), interviews were carried out at home at three points during pregnancy. In the first interview, women were asked to look back to their previous low birthweight pregnancy and asked, 'Was there anything you felt you needed in the way of support or help during that time that you didn't have?' The replies most likely to be chosen by women from a list read out to them are shown in Table 7.3.

For their current pregnancy women were asked, 'Is there anything you think would help you get through the pregnancy better, that you do not have at the moment?' The interviewer offered a list of options (but *information from doctors* was not included). The percentages of women choosing the most popular options at the second home interview during pregnancy are shown in Table 7.4.

Table 7.4   Preferences of women for their subsequent pregnancy after they had had a low birthweight baby. (Source: Oakley, 1991.)

Is there anything you think would help you get through the pregnancy better that you do not have at the moment?

Answers	% Yes
More continuity of care	40
Financial help	27
More sympathetic medical care	23
Help with housing	17
More partner support	17

Although it is possible that missing out the option information from doctors might have made a difference to these results, it is clear that improved continuity was seen as very important by the women in this study.

Taken together these studies do show that continuity of carer matters a great deal to most women. The way that the question is asked will make a difference to the sort of result that is obtained in studies of women's views. It is striking that in the MORI survey which did not suggest categories to women, continuity, good communication and supportive care all came out as important. The only caveat that I would raise is to ensure that continuity is not seen as the *only* goal of attempts to improve the personal care that women get in childbearing.

Evaluative research

I would like to turn now to research studies which have set out to evaluate new ways of providing improved continuity of carer. Unfortunately, many evaluations that have been carried out have not been reported (Wraight, *et al.*, 1993) and few of those that have been reported have employed sufficiently rigorous methods to argue convincingly for social and clinical benefits of the various types of schemes.

One randomized controlled trial was specifically designed to test the effects of improved continuity of carer. The Know Your Midwife scheme carried out by Caroline Flint and her colleagues (Flint & Poulengeris, 1987, Flint, 1991) compared the care provided by a small team of midwives with that given in the standard way. By using a randomized controlled trial, the researchers were able to be more confident that the differences that they found were due to the team care and not due to chance factors. They found that women allocated to the small team did actually experience improved continuity of carer – this cannot always be taken for granted. They also had:

- Reduced clinic waiting times;
- Improved satisfaction with antenatal care;
- Increased feeling of control in labour;
- Increased enjoyment of labour;
- Reduced use of analgesia in labour.

In addition, randomized controlled trials which have examined improved social support for childbearing women often have an element of continuity of carer as part of the intervention. These trials are very diverse in their settings and in the details of the interventions that they test. In some cases they are applied in contexts where 'standard' care is very unsupportive. A recent review of trials of continuous (social or professional) support during labour and birth (Hodnett, 1993a) has shown some striking results. The ten trials covered by this review included varied settings and support persons, but very similar components to the intervention, such as touch, praise and encouragement. The benefits included reduced use of medication for pain relief and operative vaginal delivery, and improved five minute Apgar scores. In settings where women were not permitted their own family member or friend as a companion, there were additional benefits to continuous support including reduced chance of caesarean section. It seems likely that if the presence of a support person who has not met the women before can have these dramatic effects, then providing labouring women with the support of a familiar care-giver is likely to be just as good, if not better.

There have also been a substantial number of randomized controlled trials which have offered extra social support during high-risk pregnancy (reviewed by Hodnett, 1993b,c). In spite of good reasons to expect that the interventions might be effective (Oakley, 1992) these trials have not been successful in reducing serious clinical problems such as low birthweight. Some of the individual trials do show some social and psychological benefits but the meta-analysis which puts the results from all the trials together does not indicate that this form of intervention should be put into practice. It may be that results would be different if the intervention were more targeted and intense (Hodnett, 1993b). Some other conclusions emerge from the rather varied range of evaluative studies. First, putting a new type of care into place is not straightforward. Changes do not always turn out in the way expected by the innovators. Collaborations between clinicians and social scientists have provided details of the process of change, as well as looking at outcomes – for example, in two important studies in Scotland in the early 1980s (Hall, et al., 1985; Reid, et al., 1983).

Secondly, it is *not* clear that one-to-one care – i.e. complete continuity of carer – is preferable even if it is achievable. There could be some advantages to a scheme that involved the woman in getting to know a small group of midwives (and doctors, if appropriate). She would have access to a range of skills and personalities. She would be less likely to be disappointed if the midwife she was expecting to care for her was unavailable (Currell, 1990).

Thirdly, some of the in-depth studies suggest that just getting to know a small number of staff may not help women much if the staff attitudes are stereotyped or unsupportive (Reid, et al., 1983).

A more detailed analysis of existing research and the results of several important ongoing and planned trials of continuity of care schemes could provide much clearer guidance about the relative importance of three main facets:

(1) The relationship between woman and care-giver(s);
(2) Consistent care and advice;
(3) Supportive and respectful attitudes from care-givers.

Some basic steps to assess new maternity care schemes

Many changes in the organization of maternity care are taking place (Wraight, *et al.*, 1993). New midwifery structures have arisen partly in the context of the wider movement towards individualized care and away from task orientation, partly in response to economic constraints, and partly in order to improve the personal quality of the care provided to women and their families. Because all care has at least some power to do harm as well as good, and because maternity care is one of the most complex types of health care, it is crucial to look critically at new patterns of care. Here are some points to be considered:

- Look at what you have before you introduce change. Some new schemes have destroyed important existing elements of continuity of carer.
- Set clear goals – evaluation is difficult without clear objectives. Some team schemes have not made any explicit reference to improved continuity of carer. It is important to separate goals of the scheme that apply to women and those that apply to midwives. The targets set as a result of the report of the Cumberlege Report (1993) will be very helpful to those who wish to make their care more appropriate and accessible.
- Think about evaluation before you start the scheme. It will be difficult to persuade others of the benefits of the scheme if there is no base-line description of the service as it was running before the new system was introduced. This means that the hasty introduction of a new system of care is inadvisable. Planning some sort of more or less detailed evaluation is also very useful in helping to clarify the goals of the scheme.
- Use basic audit to assess whether the goals are being met. For example, are women seeing fewer care-givers in the course of their care? Several studies have pointed to women's disappointment when a new scheme fails to provide the promised continuity of carer.
- Adopt realistic methods of evaluation. There is no need for all changes in the organization of care to involve complex and costly evaluation. On the other hand those who initiate a change need to bear in mind the potential disadvantages of a new system as well as the likely benefits. Different research designs can provide different types of evidence about the pros and cons of alternative systems of care. Where possible any evaluations should be published so that others can benefit from the work carried out.

Chapter 8
Team Midwifery

Introduction

'We conclude that there is a strong desire among women for the provision of continuity of care and carer throughout pregnancy and childbirth, and that the majority of them regard midwives as the group best placed and equipped to provide this.

(Winterton Report, 1992)

The emphasis given to continuity of care and carer in the Winterton Report was echoed in 1993 in the Cumberlege Report, which argued that:

'Throughout her pregnancy, and most particularly during labour, the woman should be cared for by people who are familiar to her and aware of her plans for delivery.'   (Cumberlege Report, 1993)

The team midwifery model is suggested as one way in which services can be organized to enhance continuity and deliver more woman-centred care.

This chapter describes the principles and practice of this rapidly evolving form of maternity care, paying particular attention to the implications for midwives of working in teams. The chapter comprises four main sections. Following this introduction, the first part of the chapter outlines the development of the team approach and raises some key concerns. The second section describes the spread of team midwifery schemes. In the third section we highlight some of the professional and labour relations issues which have arisen. The fourth, and largest part, of the chapter is devoted to illustrating some of these issues with reference to a particular scheme.

Development of the team approach

The concept of continuity of care in midwifery is not new, but as major changes take place in the provision of maternity services across England

and Wales, pressure is mounting to replace the fragmented care now in operation in many maternity units with a type of care which will meet the needs of both consumers and professionals. It is widely believed that one of the most effective ways of achieving continuity will be to reduce the number of professional staff involved in the care of each woman, and to ensure that they work together as a team. As the Royal College of Midwives has pointed out:

'In areas with conventionally organised maternity services, a pregnant woman is likely to meet a GP, a consultant, and several different midwives during her pregnancy, when she gives birth and during the postnatal period; some women may see as many as twelve professionals during this period.'   (RCM, 1991)

Although there is no single accepted definition of team midwifery, the central idea is that a small team of midwives takes responsibility for the majority of care of individual women, before, during and after the birth of their children.

Team midwifery is seen as a partial solution to providing continuity while accommodating a range of practical difficulties. Such practical difficulties stem from the historical development of midwifery services, terms and conditions of service, and the requirement that the NHS provides care on an equable basis.

On the question of equity, some commentators have argued that, in schemes where only selected women are cared for by teams of midwives, it is apparent that there is a two-tier service. In some cases the charge of exclusivity has led, in part at least, to a scheme's demise.

The institutionalization of birth from the late 1940s led to the growth of hospital-based midwifery services, and in turn to the increased numbers of, and specialization of midwives. This specialization has continued to the extent that midwives' skills in some areas are said to have become 'compartmentalized' (Curran, 1986). The separation of hospital and community midwifery, and the further specialization of hospital midwives does not fit easily with the concept of team midwifery, in which each midwife is capable of providing 'total midwifery care'.

It has been suggested that in order to provide a full named midwife service, each midwife would either have a smaller workload (in terms of numbers or complexity) than the current national average caseload, or would have to work longer hours and be highly flexible. Most NHS midwives are contracted to work $37\frac{1}{2}$ hours per week, sometimes with additional on-call responsibilities. Enhanced continuity would demand greater flexibility in terms of shifts, input and levels of responsibility than the widespread interpretation of national conditions and grading criteria suggests.

The Cumberlege Report (1993) noted that midwifery group practices operating outside the NHS demonstrate high quality practice and the most complete continuity of care, but that their costs may be higher than conventionally organized care. Costs depend on the model of team midwifery adopted, the grades of midwives involved, and on the amount of updating and re-training required.

To date there is no definitive evidence that team midwifery is more or less cost effective than other forms of maternity care. Formal and informal evaluations of team midwifery schemes have generally reported more advantages than disadvantages (for example, reductions in analgesia, episiotomies and length of labour, and increased take up of breastfeeding) but in the absence of detailed cost information and reliable quality and outcome indicators, it is difficult to draw firm conclusions about cost effectiveness.

Mapping team midwifery

An early attempt to introduce team midwifery was tried in Scotland in the late 1960s (Auld, 1968) but failed to demonstrate any improvement in patient satisfaction. A number of team schemes were set up in Wales in the mid-1970s, for example Machynlleth in 1974, Builth Wells and Newton in 1975 and Llandrindod Wells in 1976. These early schemes were predominantly small in terms of the number of deliveries, but covered both hospital and community care.

Interest in reorganizing midwifery services increased in the mid 1980s as dissatisfaction with conventional care grew. Much of the current interest in team schemes was prompted by publication of *Maternity Care in Action* (Maternity Services Advisory Committee, 1982) and by the St George's Know Your Midwife scheme, a randomized controlled trial conducted between 1983 and 1985 (Flint & Poulengeris, 1987; Frohlich & Edwards, 1989).

The spread of team midwifery has been rapid. By 1992, over a third of the 269 maternity units in England and Wales reported that they were operating some form of team midwifery scheme (Wraight, *et al.*, 1993). Three-quarters of these schemes were set up since 1987, and almost half in the last two years. In addition, a further 25 pilot schemes are currently operating. It should also be noted that a comparatively large number of schemes have been abandoned. More than a quarter of the team schemes set up in 1990 had been discontinued by 1991. The reported reasons for this range from inadequate staffing, problems with deployment, lack of commitment from midwives and from consultants, to failure to increase continuity of care.

Although the theme of improving continuity of care remains central to all these schemes, the practical implementation of the team approach varies considerably in virtually every aspect – size of teams, clinical areas covered, midwives included, allocation of women.

Team care may be applied to part or all of the service. For example, if team midwifery has been introduced in the hospital but not in the community, then the team approach will be operated alongside a more conventional service in the community. Alternatively, two approaches may co-exist where team care is offered to some mothers but not others.

In over half of the units team midwifery was confined solely to hospital care (31) or community care (24). Teams of midwives providing both hospital and community care were reported in 45 units. The latter may be organized in several ways. They may operate independently or hospital and community teams may operate in parallel. Examples of truly integrated services, in which the same midwives provide care whether the woman is at home or in the maternity hospital (that is, they follow their caseload), are still comparatively rare.

Industrial relations and professional issues

The Cumberlege Report notes:

'Making continuity of carer a reality will require a substantial degree of flexibility from midwives and their managers. Some midwives will welcome the opportunity to develop their skills more fully, and will be able to adjust their personal lives so that they can be available when a woman needs them. For other midwives this will not be the case'.

(Cumberlege Report, 1993)

The development of the team approach raises a number of professional and industrial relations issues for midwives, some of which are briefly examined in this section. These issues include:

- The role of part-time midwives;
- The deployment of core midwives;
- Changing shift patterns, flexible hours, on-call arrangements;
- Professional and career development;
- Clinical grading.

The size and composition of teams varies considerably. In some units there are nine or more teams with perhaps five or six midwives in each. In others, there may only be two teams with 16 or more midwives in each team. In general we can say that hospital-based schemes have a smaller number of teams but that the teams themselves are larger and that over half the qualified midwives are likely to be graded E. In contrast, community schemes tend to have a larger number of small teams, staffed by G grade midwives.

Such differences raise questions about the general applicability of the clinical grading structure to team midwifery. The issue of the deployment of grades lower than G for midwives working part or all of their time in the community is the most obvious example, but there are other complications. For example, hospital team members graded E provide total care to women during their span of duty. There can be no doubt that in some units the role of E grades have fundamentally changed – not only are Es called upon to undertake duties they would not previously have been expected to do, but there are occasions when an E grade is left in charge of an entire area (for the team) and has to organize absence cover.

The issue of midwives who choose (or are allocated) to remain in the 'core' providing support to community and hospital-based teams also arises. From one perspective retaining a core of midwives presents an opportunity for midwives reluctant to work in teams to continue practising in the unit. However, this in turn raises the prospect of two separate workforces and two tiers of midwives, with different grading, and different opportunities for development. Some core midwives are resentful of what they see as a secondary role, giving care only as a last resort when a team member is not available.

While the number of contractual hours for team midwives has not changed, and is in line with Whitley guidelines, there is a demand for considerable flexibility within that number of hours. For the most part, hospital based teams continue to work (sometimes modified) shift patterns. In the community, and in areas with an integrated service, midwives have had to become more flexible in terms of the hours they actually work. In some areas on call systems have been set up to cover nights, and in others the hospital provides a central advice service. The frequency and length of on call requirement has been reported to be the biggest single difficulty of working in team midwifery (Stock & Wraight, 1993).

Clearly on call working will be difficult for many part-time staff who may have chosen working hours to suit their personal circumstances. Practical difficulties, disruption to domestic arrangements and additional costs of child care may dissuade part-time midwives from working in teams. Most managers agree that in principle part-time working conflicts with continuity of carer, and continuity of care. However, there is also general recognition that in a service provided largely by women for women, part-time working must be accommodated if post career-break returners are not to be discouraged. In some schemes, part-time staff are viewed as a valuable asset, who may be available to do 'top up' hours. In other schemes the use of such staff is extremely limited.

Career development and role definition within a team structure undoubtedly pose difficulties. In small teams all midwives ostensibly do the same things, and carry the same responsibilities. Where roles are not clearly differentiated, and grading criteria are unclear, the problems become potentially more pernicious. If continuity of care, delivered through team midwifery, is to become the dominant model, then there must be scope to facilitate development within teams.

Midwives working in units with team midwifery highlight a number of costs and benefits to such schemes. Chief amongst the benefits are the personal and professional opportunities which arise from being able to use all of their skills, the high levels of peer support, and increased morale and job satisfaction which are said to result. The costs of team midwifery include the need to work more flexible hours, the need to occupy roles generally attracting higher grading, and the fact that roles within teams are often poorly differentiated, but differentially rewarded. Further, greater continuity may conflict with the ability to work part-time, to work preferred shifts, or to work in a preferred area.

Team midwifery in practice

This section describes the development of one team midwifery scheme, illustrating some of the issues outlined above.

The unit has an annual caseload of approximately 6000 births, drawn from a large geographical area and a diverse mix of client groups. It operates with a total midwifery workforce of approximately 125 whole time equivalent (WTE) hospital midwives supported by five WTE nurses and 36 WTE auxiliaries, and 64 WTE community midwives.

In 1987 the midwifery service began to look at a team structure as a means by which to increase choice for mothers, and improve continuity of care. At the time the unit served some peripheral units and a small general practitioner scheme, but the dominant model was consultant care. The unit suffered recruitment and retention problems, and there was a feeling that midwives were not able to utilize their skills effectively.

The unit has taken an evolutionary (rather than big bang) approach to the introduction of team midwifery. Team midwifery started in 1988 when midwives were invited to join small hospital-based teams providing midwife-led care in low risk pregnancies under the home-from-home scheme. Midwives were sceptical initially and very few came forward. It was through the dedication and commitment of these volunteers that two home-from-home teams developed at the unit. The success of the home-from-home scheme convinced the managers and midwives that the team approach could be extended.

Geographically-based teams were set up in 1990 and hospital teams were implemented in January 1991. Midwifery care is now provided by nine teams of community midwives linked with nine teams of hospital midwives. The nine teams currently operate three variations of team midwifery described below and illustrated in Fig. 8.1.

In the first variation, two home-from-home teams provide care to women throughout the geographical area served by the unit. Home-from-home care is provided by midwives and enables mothers and

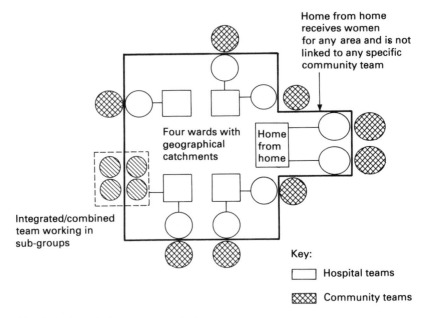

Fig. 8.1   Hospital and community team.

relatives to stay in family bedrooms close to the delivery suite before the birth.

For the remainder of the caseload there are four wards serving geographical areas within the district. Three have two consultants (in a four-tier structure), and one has one consultant. In the second variation, a team of hospital midwives is attached to each consultant, and each team provides midwifery services to a given geographical area. Hence there are seven hospital teams. Each hospital team is associated with a community team providing care for the same geographical area. Consequently there are seven sets of paired hospital and community teams each covering a geographical area.

One of these seven pairs of teams is developing the next phase, exemplifying the third variation. The hospital team and associated community teams have combined to form a team of 24. It has been recognized that this is too large a number to work as one team, and so the midwives have further subdivided into four groups of six (again, geographically based) consisting of two Gs from the community, and a G or F and remaining Es from the hospital side. The associated hospital and community teams have begun the process of orientating to each others' working areas, and an additional clinic has been set up in the community served. Eventually each midwife will provide an integrated service, and there will no longer be a division between hospital and community midwives.

Once the decision to examine the potential for hospital teams had been taken, a midwife was employed whose remit included the introduction of team-based midwifery care. A working group of midwives was set up to examine options. Midwives were invited to attend 'open forums' to put their views and discuss their concerns, and the school of midwifery was kept informed of developments. Regular progress bulletins were distributed to staff. Final proposals were put to medical and midwifery staff.

There had been some rotation of junior staff prior to teams, but many of the midwives had been working in one area of the hospital for some time (often many years) and there was a need for rapid updating. This resulted in a considerable amount of moving around, and some disruption to patient care for a short period.

The change to hospital teams was undertaken without new resources. Essentially, the total number of staff available was distributed between the teams. This resulted in an establishment of approximately eleven WTEs per team. Before teams were introduced, there had been no H grade posts in the unit (although there were I grade posts). There was also a total of 37 G grade posts, G grades having responsibility for separate areas of the unit. A total of nine H grade posts was established – one for each hospital team. This was felt to be appropriate because the team leader has 24 hour responsibility covering all hospital areas. Much of the H grade job is ostensibly concerned with management of the team, but in practice midwives report that clinical responsibilities take up much of the time they are notionally allotted for management. Team leaders take it in turns to carry the bleep for the whole of the unit.

All staff were invited to apply for H grade posts, and all posts were filled internally. The number of Gs was therefore reduced by disestablishing the posts of those who moved to H grades, and disestablishing (or in some cases changing to F) posts as they fell vacant. G grades assist the H grades, and have more responsibility for teaching. While there were previously no Fs, there is now one in each of the six teams, and a seventh in charge of the day-to-day running of the delivery suite.

There is some concern that if team midwifery results in a flatter structure, it is more likely to flatten out at E grade. Midwives of all grades felt that Es were to some extent exploited by the team approach. They felt that if a flatter structure were to work, there should be recognition of experience (rather than length of service).

The issue of grading is recognized by all concerned as a potential problem which will not go away. However there is also general acceptance that teams are here to stay, that they are the 'right way' for midwifery care to go, both for mothers and midwives. Some compromize is inevitable within the current national grading structure for midwives. The unit is soon to appoint its first E grade midwife in a developmental post to work as part of the integrated team – primarily in the community. It is likely to be an internal appointment. This is seen to exemplify the need for developmental posts below grade G if the integrated team-based approach is to become the dominant model of care.

The shift pattern was altered prior to the introduction of hospital teams, based on an analysis of workloads. Hours 'saved' are used to enable night staff to come on to the day shift to undertake an antenatal clinic. Staff are now more evenly distributed throughout the 24 hour period than previously. Staff noted that internal rotation has led to some very long work periods – midwives sometimes work consecutive shifts. Further, staff now note they are unable to leave the work area during their meal breaks.

There are two teams on each ward. When cover is required the team looks to their own part-time staff to do extra hours. Part-time staff are accommodated into teams and are seen as a useful resource as their hours can be topped up to cover for sickness absence and holidays.

Full-time staff from the team might be asked to work extra hours, and time owing is usually granted within a reasonable period. Teams also look to their sister teams on the ward for cover. When other possibilities have been exhausted bank staff are called in.

When the teams were introduced, it was made clear that the bulk of staff would have to rotate through days and nights, as well as through all areas of the hospital. However there has been compromise on this issue: some staff with sound reasons for particular preferences have been accommodated in the core staff and others have 'special' arrangements whereby they work the bulk of their time on their preferred shift. As with part-time staff these arrangements apply only as long as is necessary – that is while the special circumstances justify special treatment. All special allowances and payments for unsocial hours which were in existence before the introduction of hospital teams have so far been retained.

Midwives at the unit are unanimous that the approach taken has enhanced their job satisfaction and their professional development. They noted that rather than referring to the obstetricians as they might have done before, they are now more inclined to refer to each other. They also note that the team approach has been useful for students, who benefit from greater continuity. Students are assigned to mentors within teams for the 2–3 month duration of their stay on the unit. There have been concerns that students may not be involved in the 40 births their vocational training requires, but so far these problems have been addressed within the team structure.

Midwives believe that mothers now benefit from increased choice. The quality and continuity of information to the client has increased considerably, as has continuity of care. Continuity of carer is not guaranteed by the model of midwifery practised here, although mid-wives note there is now a 'good chance' that a mother will have met somebody from her team when she comes to deliver.

Conclusions

Given that continuity of care is the most prominent reason reported by midwifery managers for moving to team-based care, it is perhaps surprising that only half the units with teams report having a recognized caseload per team and only a third can identify the proportion of women delivered by a known midwife (Wraight, *et al.*, 1993).

More than half the units with team schemes who said that they could identify the proportion of women delivered by a known midwife, claimed that 60% or more of women knew their midwife before deliv-ery. In contrast, less than one in three deliveries was by a known midwife in units with conventionally organized care.

These figures should be interpreted cautiously. It is not known what definitions were used, how the data were collected nor the degree of accuracy that can be attributed to them. Overall, there is little general evidence that units where care is provided under team midwifery achieve higher levels of continuity of carer, although there is agreement amongst midwives that continuity of care, and quality of care, is enhanced.

The fact that so many of these schemes have been implemented in recent years demonstrates an enthusiasm among midwives to improve the standard of midwifery care. At the same time it underlines the need for careful evaluation of such changes.

Team midwifery in the UK is still in its infancy. It is not a panacea, delivering immediate solutions to the problem of providing continuity of care. There will always be arguments about the best use of resources and the need to balance quality and quantity of care within budgetary constraints. The Winterton and Cumberlege reports will have an important impact on purchaser requirements and ultimately on contracts. However, providers will not automatically be able to switch over to woman-centred care without a review of working practices, working hours, careers and compensation for midwives. Continuity cannot be delivered on the cheap.

Acknowledgements

This chapter draws on two research projects conducted by the Institute of Manpower Studies. Firstly, the mapping team midwifery project, which was commissioned and funded by the Department of Health.

Secondly, a review of industrial relations and professional issues in team midwifery, which was commissioned and funded by the Royal College of Midwives.

Part 3
Reflection on Change

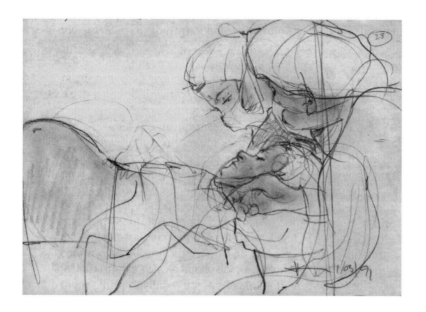

Chapter 9
Working in Practice

Introduction

The woman and her family are central to excellence in midwifery, and it is my belief that the needs of women should be a major controlling influence over professional practice. Midwives are accountable to women, who have the right to be equals in the relationship which develops between them and the midwife. In the process of putting women at the centre, midwives must be able to get to know women so that they can provide care relevant to the individual. The practice of team midwifery – where a small group of midwives provides a service for an identified group of women – seems to enable women and midwives to form relationships with each other, and in my experience, allows them to get to know each other on a deeper level than that which is possible in the traditional organization of maternity care. The purpose of this chapter is to give a personal account of how being a practitioner of midwifery within a team gave me greater independence in my practice, and to show how some of the principles described in the previous chapter can be used in the everyday work of the midwife in a new organization. All names of clients in this chapter are fictitious.

As a student midwife in 1984, my most memorable experience was to have been able to provide antenatal support and care to a woman who had been bereaved of her partner during pregnancy. It was not usual practice for the midwife to whom I was 'attached' to provide intrapartum care, but it seemed particularly important for this woman to be able to form a relationship with a midwife in pregnancy who would also be present in labour and at the birth of her child, someone who would know something of how she was feeling, her fears and wishes. When it was proposed that I be on call for her labour, she welcomed the suggestion and we were able to discuss her needs prior to labour. Support for myself was to be provided by one of the midwives on duty on the labour ward at the time.

I visited Susan at home during her pregnancy, and also saw her at her local health centre, and on these occasions we discussed her feelings surrounding her bereavement, and also her wishes for labour, in particular her fear of needles and intravenous drips. When Susan came into the hospital in labour, because she knew me, and we had talked about her loss, there was no potentially difficult introduction. Building up a relationship of trust with someone in established labour whom one had never met before, and who was also in the process of bereavement could have been very difficult, but because we already knew one another and had discussed her feelings it was not necessary for her to have to explain anything. Being well aware also of her fears, I was able to act as her advocate, expressing her concerns at a time when she was vulnerable and less able to voice them herself. Because we had built up a trusting relationship prior to labour, Susan said she felt less afraid than perhaps she would have without someone there whom she knew. For myself, I experienced a satisfaction which I had not encountered so far in my experience of midwifery, and this continued into Susan's postnatal care, as I visited her at home under the supervision of her community midwife.

Susan was the only woman during my training for whom I was able to provide care at home, in the community and in hospital. For the remaining time, and in my early experience as a qualified midwife, I worked under the traditional organization of midwifery, where the majority of care was provided by different midwives, either in the hospital or community antenatal clinics, the antenatal, labour and postnatal wards or by the community midwife at home. Women were receiving fragmented care from different midwives depending on their stage in the childbearing process, and as a learner I was not seeing the *complete* effect of midwifery care in relation to women and their families. I was experiencing either antenatal, intrapartum or postnatal midwifery practice for each woman, rather than total midwifery for the individual.

Becoming a practitioner and being *with the women*

My work with Susan had been satisfying because of the relationship we had built, and because I was able to develop a range of midwifery skills centred around one woman's experience. This seemed to make the whole picture of pregnancy and birth clearer to me as a learner. I did not have the opportunity to work with women again like this until five years later in 1989, when I was offered the chance to work as a midwife on a pilot study of a new organization of midwifery in Kidlington, Oxfordshire. The study was to explore the possibility of providing continuity of care for a group of 250–300 women and their families by a team of six midwives who would follow them from their community and homes, to hospital if necessary, and back home again. Each woman would be linked to a 'primary midwife', but she would also get to know the rest of the team, and in labour any one of the team would be on call to provide care and support.

The prospect of being able to provide women with a more satisfying childbearing experience through team midwifery was exciting. I hoped that this organization of midwifery would allow women to express their needs for pregnancy, labour and early parenting more effectively, thus allowing midwives to give them appropriate care. I looked forward to having the opportunity of using all the midwifery skills and knowledge which I had developed, up until now in a fairly piecemeal way. I had often heard the term 'practitioner' being used in relation to midwives, but so far, in my experience of being employed as a hospital midwife, I had been a practitioner of antenatal, intrapartum or postnatal care, rather than a practitioner of midwifery, being *with women* throughout their experience of childbearing.

In the process of putting women and their families at the centre of midwifery practice, and in ensuring that women receive individual and appropriate care, midwives need to be able, as far as is possible, to put themselves 'in the woman's shoes' – to have empathy with them. So, the midwife is striving to think, 'if I were *this* woman, what would I want?' In order to put oneself in someone else's position, it helps to know them quite well as a person – the way they live, their ideas, beliefs and culture – and when midwives are given the opportunity to practise in small teams, where they follow women from their homes and communities, to the place in which they give birth and then back home, they are more able to get to know women because they are seeing them regularly, and mainly on home ground. Although a midwife with good interpersonal skills can usually build up a rapport with a woman reasonably quickly, getting to know someone and building a relationship of trust takes time.

Empathy is enhanced as the woman's relationship with the team develops. The primary midwife begins the relationship with a woman, communicates her needs with the other team members, and ensures they have also had a chance to meet her, so that when it is time for the woman to give birth, whichever team midwife is on call is able to give appropriate support.

The following example helps to illustrate how the continuing relationship with the woman enhances empathy. Jean was expecting her second baby, and during her booking visit at home we discussed how she had felt following the delivery of her first child, Michael. I had been with Jean for her first labour and delivery, which had been shortly after team midwifery was introduced into the area, so we had not had a chance to get to know one another during her pregnancy. Jean had coped very well during labour, which had been long owing to the baby being in the occipito posterior position. She had managed to control her pain using Entonox. However, in spite of her being upright and in the 'all fours' position most of the time, the baby had failed to rotate and Jean had required a rotational forceps delivery, which was performed by a doctor who had had a difficult night on call, and who seemed impatient to perform the delivery before the pudendal block became effective. The delivery was both physically painful, with an episiotomy which extended to a third degree tear, and emotionally scarring for Jean who felt guilty and inadequate, because she felt as if she had lost control of herself at the point of delivery. As the midwife present, I could not help feeling that I also had failed for not being more assertive and standing up for Jean, and angry with myself for not insisting on further analgesia being given. In the days following Michael's birth, because I was also the midwife responsible for Jean's postnatal care, I was able to allow her to talk a lot about her experience, and to remind her of how calm and controlled she had been during labour, trying to get her to focus on the positive aspects in the home and to re-establish her self esteem, as well as enabling her to go over the facts of the part which had been so traumatic. I was also able to reflect on my own actions and learn from them for the future, realizing that for Jean's benefit I should have been more assertive with the doctor at the time of delivery. (In the traditional system I would have been unlikely to have become aware of quite how the experience had affected Jean, because I might not have seen her again.)

When I booked Jean for her second pregnancy, the fact that I had already formed a relationship with her previously and had experienced first hand the effects of her first labour seemed to enhance my ability to put myself in her shoes, and understand her concerns more fully. As the pregnancy progressed I was able to develop this empathy, and when her expected date of delivery approached, we discussed her wishes for labour, and her greatest fear – losing control. I discussed her anxieties with my colleagues on the team, so that they would also be under-standing of her needs and be prepared to offer Jean the right sort of support should I not be on call when she went into labour. Jean had met the other team members during this pregnancy, and she also knew some of them from last time. She asserted that she was relieved by the knowledge that there would be someone present in labour whom she knew, and who would know her and what her worries were.

I was pleased to be woken at 3 AM when Jean went into labour. Having actually been through her previous experience with her, I felt I was going to understand her needs perhaps more fully than anyone else. Jean's words over the telephone when I answered seemed to echo my feelings – 'I'm glad it's you!'. Her contractions were every five minutes, and she wished to meet me at the hospital, as she felt her labour was well established. Whilst I was driving to the hospital, I was able to reflect again on the events of Jean's first labour, and realize some of what she must be feeling now. My main role as her supporter, as for any woman in labour, would be to help her maintain strength and confidence, in order that she would stay in control. I think that my knowledge of her as a person and our continuing relationship over a period of time positively influenced the quality of support I was able to give her.

Jean was much more confident after Amy's birth, feeling she had managed to stay in control, and that she had achieved her aims. Our continuing relationship had enabled me to have a greater empathy with Jean, keeping *her* needs central to my care and allowing her to direct my practice relating to her.

During my experience with the Kidlington team, where there were six or seven midwives, women did get to know some midwives better than others, but even just having met someone once, and knowing her as one of a working group of midwives seemed to be reassuring to women. Restricting the number of midwives in a team would help to strengthen the relationships which develop between them and their clients. As a team midwife, I felt that my ability to put myself in the woman's position when giving midwifery care was enhanced as I got to know her better, which enabled me to become more aware of clients as individuals, members of a family and a community, with social, emotional, spiritual as well as physical needs.

Knowing the consequences of care

In practising a new organization of midwifery where women are followed through the system by midwives, the consequences of midwifery care are seen directly by the midwife who has provided the care. Midwives are accountable to the families they served – accountable for both their weaknesses and their strengths. I have found in team midwifery practice that one has a greater sense of accountability to women as individuals. In my opinion this is probably because one is going to see them again, and feels a greater responsibility for their well-being as a friend, as well as in a professional way.

The continuing relationship also seems to help the professional development and continuing education of the midwife, in that she sees the end result of decisions she has made. For me, this was particularly helpful when developing a new skill, such as suturing the perineum after delivery. I was taught the skill of perineal repair in the traditional system of midwifery, whilst working on the delivery suite. Whenever possible, I would try to follow the women up by visiting them on the postnatal ward prior to their transfer home, in an attempt to reflect upon my practice. However, this was difficult because often the women had already gone home before I could get to see them, and if I did see them, it was usually only in the first two or three days after delivery, at a very early stage in the healing process. I therefore had to rely on feedback from the community midwife if I was to know of any problems which were occurring as a direct result of my practice, or indeed to find out whether I was being successful in this area of practice. When I began following women through the system on a regular basis in the practice of team midwifery, I was able to see the direct consequences of my care, and where my practice was successful, I felt satisfied and my confidence was increased. If there was a problem, I knew about it and was able to seek further teaching from my mentor in this area, which enhanced my ability for future practice, enabling me to adjust my technique for the benefit of the women I was working with.

When one is seeing the consequences of care and how this may affect the future happiness of the families involved, I believe this gives a much greater sense of responsibility. The midwife sees a woman again for her postnatal care, and probably in the health centre a few months later when she happens to be visiting her family doctor or the baby clinic, or in the locality when out on visits, and perhaps for another pregnancy in the future, so it seems even more important to make every effort in helping a family to feel satisfied than perhaps in the traditional system where one will probably never see the family again. Where results are successful and families are happy with their care, the midwife feels a real sense of satisfaction and achievement as a major influence in the outcome. Midwives are more able to reflect on their actions because they are seeing the consequences of their care, and if this means they need to develop a particular area of practice, they become quickly aware of their own learning needs.

Becoming a team midwife and following individual women through the process of pregnancy, labour and the postnatal period helped to enhance my comprehension of the normal process of childbearing and the wide variations from the norm which can occur. For example, my understanding of the process of normal labour became clearer as I regularly cared for women from the early stages of labour, often at home, through to delivery in hospital or at home. My previous experience was that I would either admit women in early labour and care for them until the next shift change, or take over the care of women already in labour from the previous shift. It was unusual, particularly with primi gravidae, to experience the total labour of an individual from start to finish. As a team midwife, following women's labours throughout, my confidence in women and the ability of their bodies to succeed, increased.

Making clinical decisions

Decision making is an integral part of midwifery practice, and in my experience of the traditional organization of midwifery and team midwifery, I have found that where one is able to give continuity of care, decision making can be more effective from both the midwife's and the client's points of view. Because a closer relationship is built with the woman, the midwife understands her needs as a person and is able to work *with her* in making decisions.

The midwife is able to develop an ability to make decisions through seeing the direct results of previous decisions and reflecting upon them. Thus it is easier to assess the quality and accuracy of a professional judgement. Midwives are human, and occasionally they may make errors of judgement in their clinical decision making. In team midwifery, because they are seeing the consequences of care, midwives are not only able to learn from their mistakes but also find it possible, because of the relationship they have formed with the woman, to be open and discuss with her what should have been different. This may also help women to understand and accept bad outcomes more readily.

Decision making is less easily transferable to others when continuity of care is being given, because I think midwives feel more directly accountable to women they know, and who they are going to be seeing again. I also believe that midwives may work harder and spend more time in achieving good results through appropriate decisions for women when they are going to be seeing them again. Even if this seems to be initially time consuming, in the long run the midwife's time is managed more effectively, and the mother probably feels more supported by having time spent with her when she needs it most. If a woman is having problems with breastfeeding her baby, I might decide to visit her for each feed today, because during the antenatal period we discussed her feelings of inadequacy having failed to establish breastfeeding with her first baby, and I know how important it is that she gets it right this time. Also, if I can increase her confidence during the day, she is less likely to need to call me in the middle of the night, so I may also benefit from a good night!

With continuity of care it is easier to accept responsibility for making decisions, because one will be seeing a woman again. For example, when I was allocated to work on a postnatal ward as a hospital midwife, it was sometimes difficult to decide whether a mother and baby were fit for transfer home. Maybe there was some concern that the baby was beginning to show signs of jaundice, or the perineum was not healing very well, both *potential* rather than actual problems. Of course, she would be visited at home the following day by her community midwife who would be perfectly able to take the appropriate action, but for myself I found it difficult to accept responsibility to make the decision to send her home. Perhaps I would suggest she stayed one more night so we could review the situation in the morning. This might have all sorts of consequences both for the woman and for the organization. Perhaps she had other children at home who she was missing, or perhaps the extra night in hospital would have a negative effect on her overall satisfaction with the birth experience. For the hospital, there was the cost of the additional night's stay and of any medical intervention which might be carried out, perhaps unnecessarily. As a team midwife, when I knew I would be seeing the woman again myself, I found it easier to make the decision to transfer her home, because I was not having to pass on the responsibility of *possibly* needing to refer her to a doctor, to someone else. Even if I was going on holiday the following day, I felt confident in the knowledge that my colleagues on the team would take over in the same philosophy of care, as I could directly communicate my concern to them. Another advantage of knowing the woman, and her home circumstances was that I knew whether she had the facilities at home to be able to keep per perineum spotlessly clean to aid healing. If I knew she lived in hostel accommodation with shared bathroom, and after discussion with her we decided she should stay in hospital, then it would be an *appropriate* decision.

Sometimes the midwife has to be her client's advocate in getting a medical decision made in her best interests. For example, Valerie's general practitioner arranged for her to visit the consultant obstetric clinic at the beginning of pregnancy because her first baby was born by caesarean section. Valerie went along hoping that a decision would be made regarding whether she would be having another abdominal delivery, or a trial of labour this time, so that she could begin to prepare herself mentally for the event. It was not routine for the team midwife to attend hospital appointments with women, because of the time involved and the difficulty of co-ordinating this. Women had a booking history taken in their own homes with their primary team midwife, and they then went to the consultant unit to see an obstetrician if necessary. Valerie attended her appointment, but she found it difficult to assert her needs and ask questions in the stress of the busy hospital clinic. She had been given some information and was asked to think about what she would like to do, but came away confused and uncertain, and disappointed that no clear decision was made. At her next antenatal appointment with her midwife in the health centre, she felt better able to voice her needs. The midwife was able to arrange to go with her to visit the consultant obstetrician with a clearer idea of what Valerie needed to know, and to ensure that the decision which was made was right for her and her family, and that she felt involved and informed in the process. It seemed that Valerie was given strength by being able to build up a relationship with a midwife who was able to act as her advocate, and she was able to approach the rest of her pregnancy with greater confidence. The fact that she also knew the midwife who was to be present in the operating theatre at the baby's birth seemed to complete the picture and add to the satisfaction of both the family and the midwives involved.

Using peer support and peer review

In working as a team midwife, close relationships are developed amongst team members, and this provides a safe environment for individual midwives to air anxieties or uncertainties about practice, without fear of criticism. If a particularly difficult decision has to be made, discussion within the team allows more avenues to be explored than perhaps would be if one was making the decision alone.

The team provides support if a midwife finds a particular area of practice difficult, and enables her to explore ways of dealing with the problem and move forward. This peer review benefits the team as well as the individual, because the team as a whole gains knowledge and practice is enhanced. My experience of peer review within the team was that it worked particularly well for supporting and encouraging good practice amongst colleagues, but was more difficult to use in situations where unhelpful, or unfavourable practice was to be discouraged. To work effectively, peer review depends on a trusting relationship between team members, because whilst it is relatively easy to give praise for strengths in a colleague, it is more difficult to deal with a situation where one's peer is seen to have a problem in a particular area of practice. However, as team midwifery seems to help one to reflect on one's personal practice, it also enables midwives to be constructive about their peers' practice. The whole team is accountable to the women it is caring for, and so it is to the whole team's advantage to deal with problems or difficulties which colleagues are experiencing. Self and peer review of performance enables individual midwives and the team as a whole to work out areas of weakness and strength in the team. In my experience many aspects could be dealt with within the team itself, using shared experience and knowledge. However, the help of a supportive manager or supervisor of midwives outside the team is required when peer review is inappropriate or difficult.

Working in a small team provides the opportunity to support and care for colleagues in difficult situations, such as when a baby dies. Caring for someone who has lost a baby is always very upsetting, but in my experience of this situation as a team midwife, where one has come to know the family well, it seems particularly difficult for the midwife to cope with because of the friendship which has developed during the pregnancy. Peer support is a great help and comfort when such a tragedy occurs. The team members are able to talk through the bereavement with one another and express their grief in a safe, understanding environment where colleagues know one another well.

In my experience of team midwifery I found that the midwives not only supported one another professionally, but cared for and supported each other personally. I had not experienced midwives caring for one another in quite the same way in the traditional organization of midwifery, where midwives are part of a much larger team and are not all able to get to know one another as well as in a smaller group working closely together.

Full utilization of midwifery skills and knowledge

As a practitioner of team midwifery, I was constantly in a position where I was using all my midwifery skills and knowledge all of the time in relation to individual women and babies. I found tremendous job satisfaction in being able to practise in this way, and my work became stimulating and challenging. I also found my knowledge of women and their needs developed because I was seeing them as whole people, members of families and the community, rather than women at one stage of pregnancy or another.

A typical on call day on the Kidlington team required midwives to use several of their midwifery skills and a great deal of knowledge in one 24 hour period. A real day on call for myself, for example, gave me the opportunity to do the following:

- Meet with colleagues to discuss and reflect on practice issues;
- Visit two postnatal mothers and babies in hospital and at home;
- Visit a woman who had been admitted to hospital the previous day because of a small antepartum haemorrhage, perform her cardiotocograph and arrange for her scan to be done;
- Visit a woman at her workplace, which was the most convenient place for her, to discuss prenatal diagnosis for Downs Syndrome;
- Give support over the telephone to a mother who was concerned that her baby might be constipated;
- Refer a woman with abdominal pain at 34 weeks of pregnancy to an obstetrician and admit her to hospital;
- Care for a woman in early labour at home, go with her to the hospital and help her through labour in the birthing pool.

This was a particularly busy day, but not unusual for an on call day, and although very tired at the end, I was able to go to bed feeling satisfied that I was really practising what I had been trained to do, using so many of my skills within one day's work.

Working in this way does mean that midwives must spend a lot of time keeping up-to-date with developments in all aspects of midwifery, which is a challenge in itself. Within the team, although the individual midwives have a responsibility to maintain and develop their own skills and knowledge, the group as a whole has a *pool* of knowledge and ability to be shared, and this is done with enthusiasm! In Kidlington the group had monthly and daily meetings where the midwives could reflect as a team on their practice and particular experiences or problems, sharing new or existing knowledge with one another, constantly aiming to improve practice in the team. If the team had a particular learning objective or a standard to be developed in a particular area, they worked together in achieving these, with the help of the team's lecturer practitioner. In this way, standards which are set are applicable to the area of practice and are flexible and responsive to the needs of the families for whom the team is caring. The standards also respect the needs of the team itself.

Satisfaction and commitment

Whilst practising team midwifery a deep sense of satisfaction came with getting to know women for who they were, not just as women having babies, but as part of a community and as part of a family. This knowledge helped me to understand their needs in a wider context, and *why* certain things were so important to them. In fulfilling the needs of the whole woman I often felt as if I was a part of the family, and became more involved with them as people than I had done previously.

Being a practitioner of team midwifery requires commitment, involvement and strength. Before I worked as a team midwife, I felt a commitment to midwifery, but when practising in this new organisation, I felt a greater commitment *to the women* I was with, and perhaps a greater sense of responsibility towards them because I knew them as friends. I also felt a greater commitment to work and to my colleagues, and was more prepared to be flexible about work than I had been when working in the traditional organization. This might mean working on a day off because a colleague was sick, or being called in the middle of the night because someone booked for a home birth had gone into labour when the midwife on call was already with a labouring woman in hospital. I was prepared to do this because it enabled women to receive care from midwives they knew, and also because caring for women who you know is very satisfying and rewarding.

From employee to practitioner

During my experience of team midwifery I was able to move a step closer towards a position of being an independent practitioner of midwifery. I felt more responsible for my work and a greater accountability for the care I gave and the decisions I made with women. Although I sometimes found team midwifery difficult and often demanding and tiring, my work was more satisfying than I had previously experienced because I was using all my skills, and because I was more able to give individual and appropriate care to women who I had got to know. The fact that the team were given responsibility for organizing their own caseloads and way of working gave greater independence, and although practising within the NHS, I felt less like an employee and more like a practitioner who was responsible for my own actions and thus less dependent on a large organization. In allowing midwives to practise in this way where they feel a greater responsibility and accountability towards the women they are with, not only do women receive care appropriate to their needs, but also the midwife is able to move closer towards a goal of becoming an independent practitioner in her own right.

Chapter 10
Teaching in Practice

Introduction

In Britain two reforming movements are affecting the profession of midwifery. One is the change from a ward-based approach. The other is a move of pre-registration midwifery education to higher education, that is to university level. In this chapter I describe the changes as they happened in Oxford, starting in the late 1980s, the historical background to these changes, and how my work as a practitioner and teacher within the Oxford City Team is organized. In Oxford the change in practice and education was intentionally simultaneous, based on the ideals laid down by the Oxfordshire District Health Authority that education for all students of both nursing and midwifery should be at degree level, and that education should be based upon a foundation of excellence in practice.

An important part of this strategy was the creation of lecturer practitioner posts, which were filled by individuals who had a formal teaching role, but who were also truly practitioners. They developed practice not only through leadership and role modelling, but also through authority over standards in clinical practice. The position of the lecturer practitioner within the teams is a very important one. The lecturer practitioner is the teacher who brings the ideals of the classroom into practice, but those ideals themselves are informed by the reality of everyday practice. Working with the students in practice, and taking real life experience of practice into higher education can have a powerful effect on education. It is within the midwifery teams that students, the midwife practitioners of the future, will experience the practice which forms the future. Furthermore, the team approach is seen as an organization which supports the ideals of practice reflected in the theory within the degree programme. The midwifery degree programme in Oxford, which is direct entry (you do not have to be a registered nurse to get into it), was the first undergraduate programme in midwifery to be established in Britain.

131

Changes in the maternity services

Midwives have traditionally passed on their knowledge, skills and experiences to each other in order to improve the care offered to mothers and babies, and their families.

According to Cowell & Wainwright (1991), since 1881, when the Matron's Aid Society was formed, midwives have worked hard to improve standards of midwifery practice. Dame Rosalind Paget was instrumental in improving training and petitioning Parliament for the registration of midwives, which resulted in the 1902 Midwives Act.

More recently, government reports have been published which have had a profound influence upon the provision of maternity services. The organizational arrangements have, in turn, affected clinical practice and the role and responsibilities of the midwife. This, inevitably, has affected the education of student midwives.

The beginning of the reorganization of the maternity services from community to hospital-based care occurred as a result of recommendations made by the Cranbrook Committee (Ministry of Health, 1959) which recommended the provision of sufficient maternity beds for an average 70% institutional confinement rate). The resulting increase in hospital deliveries from 15% in 1955 to 80.8% in 1968 (Currell, 1990) necessitated the provision of more maternity beds. Much hospital building took place in the 1970s and the hospital birthrate gradually rose to around 99%.

In response to the need for additional maternity beds, modern maternity units were built. These centralized facilities, particularly for women with complications of pregnancy and existing medical disorders, included facilities for neonatal care. The result was a more medical approach to care.

Families living in the more rural areas were cared for locally by general practitioners and community midwives but as small maternity units were closed they had to travel to the main maternity hospital for delivery. This inevitably caused an increase in fragmentation of care for the families using the services as they were cared for by both community and hospital staff.

The 1974 reorganization of the maternity and midwifery services resulted in midwives working in either hospital or the community. In hospital, midwives were allocated to the antenatal clinic, delivery suite, antenatal or postnatal wards. The allocation of midwives to clinical areas which separated antepartum, intrapartum and postpartum care contributed to the erosion of the role of the traditional midwife using the full range of midwifery skills. It also further increased the number of midwives providing care for each woman and her family.

Changes in education

Changes in the organizational structure and culture of practice influence education and training of midwifery students. Prior to moves into higher education, students undergoing the eighteen month post-registration midwifery training were allocated to each clinical area for a number of weeks' experience both in the hospital and in the community. Student midwives and student nurses were taught by midwives in the different clinical areas. Midwifery tutors were responsible for teaching students mainly in the classroom but with sessions of clinical teaching.

One of the difficulties in visiting the clinical area was that the midwifery tutor was generally only able to spend a limited period of time with the student and consequently the care received by women was fragmented. There were other implications in that tutor and student were not exposed to the pressures on the workload by extraneous factors such as emergencies, or interruptions from enquiries or visitors which made the provision of care more difficult for the ward staff. There was also some resentment that the midwifery tutor, providing care for a short period, did not seem to have the same degree of responsibility as the ward staff for the woman's care.

Midwifery tutors had little influence over ward philosophy, policies and practices or the development of the learning environment. These were considered to be the responsibility of the midwifery sister in charge of the clinical area.

In the late 1980s many maternity units started trying to address the dichotomy between service provision and education.

In 1989, as a result of the partnership between Oxford Brookes University (formally Oxford Polytechnic) and Oxfordshire District Health Authority, the four year direct entry degree in midwifery commenced (Page & Healey, 1990). Nursing and midwifery practitioners, managers and educators worked together to develop the curriculum for the degree programme which replaced the existing eighteen month post-registration midwifery training.

The education team for the Midwifery Field (The Field of Study) consists of lecturers and lecturer practitioners. The role of the lecturer practitioner developed from the commitment to reduce the gap between education and practice (Champion, 1992). A number of lecturer practitioner posts were created in several clinical areas both in hospital and in the community.

Simultaneously a Midwifery Development Committee was formed. This provided a forum for midwives representing all parts of the midwifery service both within the John Radcliffe Maternity Unit and the surrounding community. The committee met regularly, and continues to do so. The aims are to examine the organization of midwifery services with a view to improving care for mothers and their families and to increase professional development opportunities for midwives. One working group began the development of community-based team midwifery.

In 1989 the first team of midwives was formed in the Kidlington area of Oxfordshire (Watson, 1990). The lecturer practitioners were involved in the organization and creation of the team, including the discussions with all members of the primary health care teams in Kidlington. They were also involved in the selection and appointment of the team midwives. In 1991 a second team was formed. This team provides care for the mothers registered with four general practices in the Wheatley, Headington and Cowley areas of Oxford.

Currently each team has a lecturer practitioner who is responsible for three main areas: education and the learning environment; practice; and management including budgetary control. The ratio of lecturer time to practice time varies between lecturer practitioners but in the team overall is 0.4 lecturer to 0.6 practice. This is because it is necessary to be in clinical practice regularly to provide care as a primary midwife for a designated caseload, and to maintain regular contact with members of the team. It is more difficult to provide continuity of care when working part-time as a practitioner and achievement of this requires a certain amount of flexibility.

Lecturer practitioners vary in their professional background and experience. Some have more teaching experience and have had to update aspects of their clinical practice. This has been beneficial for them – to experience again the feeling of being a learner in an unfamiliar environment. Others are experienced clinicians but have relatively recently acquired a teaching qualification. This encourages the sharing of experience and learning from each other. Regular meetings together is an important source of support.

Responsibility within the team

The team has, as far as possible, a non-hierarchical structure. All members of the team including the lecturer practitioner have worked together to formulate a shared philosophy. The midwives make decisions about the organization of the team as well as about practice. Each member of the team has a special responsibility for a particular aspect of organization, for example, the duty rota, or collection of statistical data.

Each member of the team is at a different stage of personal and professional development. The strength of a small group of midwives is in caring for each other and the continual sharing of skills and experiences. Team members help each other to reflect on practice, and through this are able to influence practices and policies.

Experiencing good practice is fundamental to the education of student midwives and opportunities for students to experience practice with midwives using the full range of skills is vital. Students are allocated to a primary mentor who gives guidance and support through the learning experiences. Students experience the support and caring attitude of midwives and feel it gives them confidence and enhances their ability to learn. The team midwives and lecturer practitioner work together to ensure the clinical learning environment is suitable for the students so that their learning is of high quality.

There are, of course, other team or group systems which provide an effective learning environment for students. The key to their success is in the restriction of numbers of midwives, six to eight seems to be the optimum number from our experience. Others recommend no more than six and ideally fewer (Wraight, *et al.*, 1993; Cumberlege Report, 1993).

Authority over standards, policies and resources

Working as one of the team enables the lecturer practitioner to gain first-hand knowledge of standards of midwifery practice within the group of midwives as well as within the midwifery service as a whole. The setting and monitoring of standards is an important part of the team's professional responsibilities.

The team midwives work in all the clinical areas both in hospital and the community. It is therefore necessary to be aware of the policies of all areas. Policies affecting specific aspects of team care are formulated by the midwives of both teams, for example, the policies regarding six hour discharge following delivery, and frequency of both antenatal and postnatal visits.

Effective communication between the team midwives and hospital staff is essential as well as those with members of the primary health care teams. The midwives have primary responsibility for particular general practitioners and the women registered with them.

There has to be a real commitment within the team to meet daily in order to discuss the clinical care. Once the daily distribution of work has taken place midwives work predominantly on their own or, during term time with a student midwife. The team midwives also have regular planning meetings and social gatherings.

Each team (six whole time equivalents) cares for 300 women and their families. This has the advantage that midwives use the full range of their midwifery skills, regularly seeing women during pregnancy, labour and the postpartum periods in hospital, the health centre or the woman's home.

Allocation of midwifery students to community-based midwives enables them to experience continuity of care and carer. Seeing the woman in the context of her home and family helps the student to identify a wide range of issues to consider when planning midwifery care. It also makes experiences more meaningful and memorable.

Continuity of care can achieve the early identification of problems and therefore prompt referral for the appropriate advice, treatment or help. Tailoring and channelling care for those women who need social, physical or psychological support means more economic use of resources in these days of financial constraints.

It is important to monitor the long-term effects of care on individuals, families and the communities served. Obstetric outcomes, infant feeding, and the effect of the experience of the maternity services on families are all evaluated.

Having responsibility for the budget is an essential part of the managerial responsibility of the lecturer practitioner within the team. It is difficult to cost the team midwifery service accurately as the midwives provide care in a wide range of settings both in hospital and in the community. There are advantages to the budget being divided between the various wards, departments and groups of midwives of the maternity service. It develops a sense of responsibility, and encourages ideas for making savings or keeping within the budget. Maternity leave has created the greatest difficulty in keeping within the team budget.

The lecturer practitioner has primary responsibility for a defined caseload which is an important aspect of the role. It increases credibility with other practitioners within the team, in the clinical areas and with other disciplines. Experiencing the reality of clinical practice is important in being able to review organization and quality of care. It also has an effect on the relationship with students both when working in the clinical areas and in the classroom.

Sessions in the classroom include discussion and reflection upon management of various clinical situations. Students value the opportunity to analyse them in a supportive environment. It is an advantage if the lecturer practitioner is familiar with both the physical and social learning environment so that all aspects of a situation can be realistically explored.

In the present climate of change in the NHS there is a great deal of anxiety and uncertainty, and a tendency to feel that change is not always for the better. There is an element of resistance to the adult-centred approach to learning. In this adult-centred approach learning is self directed and students utilize their previous personal and professional experiences as a point of departure. Students work at their own pace and identify their own learning needs through a learning contract.

The move into higher education with its adult-centred approach to learning is a change which some midwives at first find threatening. It may be difficult for them to relinquish control and to change to the role of mentor and facilitator. Preparation and support of mentors is an important part of the role of the lecturer practitioner. It is particularly challenging for mentors to change from working with midwifery students who have had a nursing background to working with students doing a direct entry midwifery course at degree level.

Managing the workload

Managing the workload of both components of the lecturer practitioner role requires flexibility. Although many aspects of the role cannot and should not be separated in order to keep education and practice together, there are certain elements of the lecturer role that can be planned.

During term time, two days of the week can be organized to be spent on activities which include meetings with the course planning team for curriculum planning, organizing and running practice-based modules, assessment of both theoretical and practical aspects of the modules and meeting with students and mentors.

The remaining three days are spent working in the team as a midwife providing antenatal, intrapartum and postpartum care with primary responsibility for a defined caseload. Team meetings, discussions about policies and practices, and developing the learning environment are included on these practice days.

During vacations there is slightly more flexibility to review long term plans, and evaluate progress. Discussions with lecturer practitioners in other areas provide valuable opportunities to examine other ways of working. The freedom to be able to develop the role to suit the particular clinical area is invaluable.

Reflection in practice

Reflective practice is an integral part of the degree programme. Supported by the work of Schön (1991) on the nature of professional practice, and Benner (1984), who examined the nature of developing expertise in nurses, the course planning team adopted a reflective practice model of professional education (Champion, 1992). Although there are many midwives who naturally reflect on practice, reflection is a skill which can and should be developed. Lecturers, lecturer practitioners, mentors and students all develop skills of reflection and reflective practice both through keeping reflective diaries and through discussion.

Working within a small team or group of midwives caring for an identified caseload provides a natural forum for regular discussions about practice. Reflection encourages a questioning nature which is positive and constructive and motivates practitioners to examine and evaluate their own practice and that of others. Opportunities for discussion between midwives is vital as they deliver care itself mainly on their own.

A daily review of care planned with clients takes place between the midwives on duty for that day. Planning the most appropriate care for each woman and, where possible, taking advice from the most skilled midwife has many advantages. It enables those present to learn, in a supportive atmosphere, from their own and other midwives' experience. This is particularly beneficial to students who participate in the process and learn from it. It also allows other resources, from the literature or other professionals, to be explored and utilized. It enables the client to have maximum benefit from the care. Van Manen (1991) describes this as anticipatory reflection.

Team midwifery, or any system which has continuity of care, also enables both midwives and students to learn directly from the consequences of their care. This not only includes care given during a current pregnancy, but as many of the mothers are cared for by the same midwives in subsequent pregnancies there is a valuable opportunity to reflect upon long term care of the family. This gives the midwives a freedom to try out a range of alternative practices and evaluate the results. The mothers play an important part in providing feedback on the care provided.

Students registered with the midwifery programme are allocated to midwife lecturers or lecturer practitioners who, as their professional tutors, guide and support them through the modular course. From the first, midwifery students are allocated to midwife mentors and observational visits and this gives them an opportunity to experience the realities of midwifery. Students are encouraged to keep a reflective diary setting down their feelings and thoughts about situations they encounter. They are excited and enthusiastic about any practical contact and it is at this time that the midwife can act as a role model and help the student keep a balance between reality and idealism.

Some will be keen to become involved in practice immediately whilst others will wish to remain observers. It is important for the experience to be student-led, respecting students' decisions and encouraging development at their own pace.

The reflective diary is a private and confidential means of working through issues. Some students bring the reflective diary for the mentor to read. The diary may form the basis for mentor and student to analyse situations at another time. It is equally useful for the midwife to have the student's perspective on events that have occurred. It is beneficial to look back at written evidence of reflection and realize that progress has been made and change has occurred. It also forms the basis for planning the direction for the future.

Students evaluate the organization and effectiveness of each module throughout the course. This includes evaluation of lecturer practitioners as module leaders, and as facilitators of learning in both the classroom and clinical settings. Many students appreciate the fact that the lecturer practitioners understand and experience the positive and negative aspects of midwifery practice and are in touch with the current realities of the learning environment.

Teaching in practice is aimed at bringing together the ideal and the real. It provides opportunities to improve standards of practice enabling good practice itself to be the focus of the student's education. Through the work of the lecturer practitioner in the midwifery team, the teacher of midwifery is able to practise within an organization which allows her a full professional role, and thus help the student, the practitioner of the future, prepare for this new style of practice. Both teacher and student practise to the full using all of their skills and abilities, with a focus on good care for the childbearing woman and her family.

Chapter 11
Seeking Effective Practice:
The Work of the Clinical Leader

Introduction

Over the last few decades midwifery has become a workforce organized from a central focus, often the hospital, and has been hierarchically arranged and controlled. Moving to group practices is not only a change in the pattern of the midwifery service, but also reflects a new philosophy of care and the need for a different style of management. The clinical leader taking forward this innovation, the development of small teams or group practices, occupies a position quite unique to midwifery management. This leader is crucial to the success of the innovation, because it is this person who is at the cutting edge, who ensures that the vision, the policies and aims of the project are actually put into practice. It is this leader, who struggles with the task of ensuring that where ideas and ideals meet the rough road of every day life, they are not twisted, compromised, or trodden down on the well worn paths of daily routine, attitudes and systems. The work requires hanging onto the vision while working through the complex and everyday details of the present system. It also requires persistence and effective communications to help turn around systems and routines which do not support the innovation.

The clinical leader or the project leader is required to work comfortably at all levels of the organization, being an integral part of the grass roots of midwifery practice while also working comfortably and effectively with those at the executive level. In general these leaders tend to be comparatively young, and are not always a part of the established management hierarchy.

Thus, many of the experiences are new, and the ability to learn quickly, to be quick-thinking, are essential. Commitment to the ideas being put into practice helps, because the role is not an easy one, and there will be many detractors of the change. This chapter is based upon our individual experiences of setting up team midwifery and group practices in midwifery. It is intended as a guide for all those who have asked what we did and how we did it. It might be that some processes and experience are relevant only to the areas in which we practised. But when we met and discussed how to write this chapter we were struck by the similarities in the experiences that we both encountered, despite four years between the two schemes. It became increasingly apparent during our discussions that both care schemes were underpinned by the same vision, guiding principles and ideas that later built the foundation of the new midwifery service.

We have both been faced with many challenges and have experienced many ups and downs during the process and implementation of change in midwifery practice. Throughout our experience we have realized that whatever the vision you are working towards, the process, style and implementation will vary according to the differing needs of the organization and population you are working with. Despite this, it is vital to remember that effective woman-centred care can take place anywhere if the vision and guiding principles are clarified at the outset. We hope you will find our experiences helpful as a guide when making change in your own area and by sharing what happened to us we offer both support and inspiration.

The role of clinical leader

Central to the success of change in midwifery practice within an organization is the role of the clinical project leader who by definition can be described as a leader, manager, clinician, change agent and who might also be a supervisor of midwives. The clinical leader is at the sharp edge of the change, responsible for moving forward the new organization of care and for translating the vision into reality. The clinical leader also has the responsibility to work alongside, guide and support other midwives towards the new style of practice.

This enabling and supportive approach is in stark contrast to much of traditional midwifery management in Britain, where the practice of individual midwives is controlled by, and sometimes policed by the senior midwife. Here, the clinical leader enables the midwives to practice, through quite consciously giving midwives the authority and power to 'run' their practice, while supporting them in developing skills, setting their own standards, and providing moral and practical support.

The journey towards achieving the vision is not easy, therefore it is essential that the clinical leader also has support within the organization, from the conception of the vision to the delivery of the service itself. Following appointment, the clinical leader needs to identify a supportive network through professional and administrative colleagues within the organization, and through links with other midwives undertaking similar ventures elsewhere. These midwives become invaluable allies in the journey that lies ahead, offering incentive and support.

Qualities and skills

Many qualities and skills are required because the role is demanding. But, as with any challenging work, many skills and abilities will be developed within the role, particularly with the right support. Knowledge of your own strengths and weaknesses is fundamental to successful leadership in any situation, but particularly in this type of situation, which requires much learning on the job, and fast responses to complex events. Building a support system or team who complement your strengths and weaknesses, and identifying areas for your own development, will be an integral part of your work as leader.

The key to success is to keep to the vision, work within the guiding principles and yet be flexible enough to adapt dynamically to unpredicted events, an inevitable part of such big changes. Strategic planning and project management are required, but these need to be accompanied by effective communication, diplomacy and persuasion, and political awareness. The clinical leader needs to be or at least to become street-wise politically.

The development of effective group practices requires profound and fundamental change in the system of care. It requires different and often much greater commitment on the part of the midwives involved. Such change requires that you have to take a large number of people with you. For such innovations to work, although a small number of people may take the innovation forward, there needs to be ownership by the organization as a whole. This requires the genuine commitment and involvement of many people. The clinical leader needs to value all staff and their contribution to care, and sensitivity is required throughout the change as hierarchical and traditional structures are challenged.

To lead others through such a change process requires a predominantly democratic rather than autocratic approach. At times however, directive management is required. All colleagues have a part to play in the implementation of the change in practice and no matter how small contributions may seem, recognition of such contributions leads to a degree of ownership of the change itself within the organization.

Making mistakes

Peters & Waterman (1982) emphasize that innovation often entails making some mistakes, and that organizations which are truly innovative accept these mistakes without censure. Successful innovators are involved in a complex matrix of change, which requires that many tasks are on the go at once. Inevitably a large number will succeed, but some will fail. No matter how intensive or careful the planning may be, teething problems do occur in the first few weeks and months, and some mistakes will be made. For us these teething problems included bleeps that did not go off, women who were missed by the system (due to moving into the area), forgetting to stock equipment, and midwives not arriving on the delivery suite on time. Midwives at the Centre for Midwifery Practice, Queen Charlotte's and Hammersmith Maternity Service had to get used to mobile telephones which caused a few problems in the early days of service because people were not used to them.

Everyone seems to notice these teething problems, while forgetting how commonly similar situations have occurred in the traditional systems. It can be trying for the midwives and the clinical leader when these teething problems, rather than success stories, become the focus of attention. The position of clinical leader, as for any leader bringing about change, can feel isolated at times. Focus on problems can be particularly demoralizing if support systems are not put in place. If these support systems are in place then positive outcomes can be focused upon, thus enhancing morale. We found that the clients themselves provided immense support and encouragement which in turn led to increased job satisfaction for midwives, and a belief in what they were doing and why they were doing it.

Planning and the process of change

Knowing where you are

In any process of change you need to know where you are now, where you want to go, and how you will get there. Reforming the service into group practices requires not only that the pattern of practice be changed but also that the culture of the organization be changed. Knowing and understanding the present culture is essential, in order to analyse what needs to be changed, what needs to be preserved, and where there will be support or resistance to the change.

When planning to implement change in midwifery practice from within the maternity service the clinical leader requires in-depth knowledge relating to both the local and national political environment. Morgan (1986) points out that if we examine the cultural factors that shape individuals and organizations we have a better chance of under-standing what is normal for any particular organization. We would argue that it is also healthy to question that normality prior to embarking on the development of a new service.

Even if group practices are to be implemented in one circumscribed part of the organization such fundamental change will impact on all of the support services. Understanding the cultural habits and routine working of the existing type of maternity service it is important not to consider it in isolation from all the services upon which such a fundamental change in midwifery practice impacts. For example, medical records, housekeeping and primary care, will all be affected. The impact of change in one area can spiral – making a change in one area often leads to a change in another, as people within the organization begin to question the status quo.

Knowing where you are going

The aims and objectives of the new organization of care and service delivery need to be established at the outset, defining clearly what is to be achieved. Once these aims and objectives are clear and agreed, they lead to the development of the details of the change, consultation documents, the business plan, identification of resources and the roles of particular people. The clarification of the aims and objectives in itself constitutes the early stages of consultation – hearing from users, commissioners of the service, professional groups and executives and other staff about their aspirations, concerns, and requirements. Then through a period of discussion and clarification these aims are written down and used as part of the formal process of consultation. Wide circulation and a period of consultation with key personnel enables others to understand the need for change and to become involved, and instils a sense of ownership of the change within the organization. Discussion with professional colleagues both in the hospital setting and the community is enlightening – it amazed both of us how many people were motivated to change the service, already had ideas and were willing to share them. The clinical leader is in a key position in this period of consultation to hear the genuine reactions of staff, particularly colleagues. The unique position rests on being generally unseparated from the grass roots, and therefore open to ideas and reactions from those below the middle management level, as well as those above it.

Steps on the way

The journey towards achieving the vision is made up of inter-related tasks or actions, each having their own specific importance and purpose and these are often dependent upon each other. The clinical leader is required to keep a broad vision, while ensuring that discrete, small tasks, are attended to and accomplished. This stage, when vision becomes reality is the most crucial. Remember, there is many a slip twixt the cup and the lip. The work of organizing midwives into small groups relies on many complex, often tedious tasks – for example, working out numbers of deliveries expected within a geographical area, changing all the case notes the night before the start to identify clients for the new care, working out new systems of referral, allocating families to individual midwives case loads, and many more. During the planning phase all tasks need to be monitored and reviewed and if necessary a new approach may be required.

Systematic strategic planning may be enhanced by the use of information technology and/or project management tools. However, it is important to remember such a complex change that impacts on so many cannot be totally rigid. Careful planning, targets and deadlines maintain motivation and direction, not only for the clinical leader but also for everyone involved. Despite changes in approach these targets can be maintained.

The clinical leader plays a crucial part in moving forward the development of group practices, but such a fundamental change can never be accomplished by one person working in isolation. Not only does such change require a groundswell of support from the workforce, but to succeed the change must have legitimacy and genuine support from the leaders within the organization (Kanter, 1984). The leader needs not only support and encouragement, but parallel work undertaken by colleagues at a senior level, in creating a climate for change, working with stakeholders and executives, in releasing resources, and gaining commitment.

In the Centre for Midwifery Practice the creation of one-to-one midwifery care required the work and commitment of a group of people from different levels of the organization and with different skills. The Director of Midwifery, the Professor of Midwifery, the researcher, and the lecturer practitioner for the development were all involved in moving the development forward and making it happen. Our group became known as the Action Group. Within this action group the roles and responsibilities of the key players required definition; however the lead person in the group might change according to the task or action to be undertaken and the skills that were required to achieve the deliverable. Balancing skills and experience enhances and produces strength within the group and at times can induce heated discussion. Sharing of knowledge, ideas and experience also enhances personal development and learning.

Advice

Formal advice from key members of the service or its stakeholders helps ensure stability and legitimacy in steering the innovation to implementation. A steering group might include members of community health councils, family health service authorities, public health departments, consumers, university lecturers and individuals with an interest in women's health. These individuals do not necessarily have to be in favour of the proposed change. In fact, it is useful to have individuals to continually challenge. An objective view and advice from others outside the 'inner circle' can help clarify ideas and provide a wider view of the proposed change and its impact. It is also relevant to delegate certain tasks to skilled individuals on a co-opted basis, bringing a fresh perspective to the group and thus generating and developing new ideas.

Meetings

We do not advocate meetings for meetings' sake. To be beneficial they need to be structured with a clear set of objectives so that progress can be made. Sometimes it is necessary to review the groups, and group memberships so that individuals can be invited along when their perspective is needed. All meetings should be noted or minuted as the information forms a basis for reflection and also provides evidence of progress and agreements that have been reached. In the early days of an innovation, project groups with clear tasks and deadlines are the most effective. They may be thinking groups, action groups, groups responsible for disseminating and cascading information, and so on. These groups should involve everyone within them as peers, no matter what their rank, and should encourage open and honest debate. If working well they should feel dynamic, but not always comfortable.

Many tasks need to be completed, and it is far better to have the involvement and thus investment of groups of people. For example, there might be a multi-disciplinary group working on risk assessment, on the finances, or on the consultation strategy.

Dissemination of information

Informing everyone who will be involved in and affected by the change is essential. Information may be powerful, but to hold it back can be a mistake. Formal and informal discussion is useful. Both forums can achieve different results; for example, what is said around a table can be quite different to what is said on an individual basis, perhaps in the delivery suite coffee room late at night, where there is not the same pressure to be politically correct. A newsletter with a contact number for the clinical leader is one way that any information can be shared and inviting feedback from colleagues enables their queries to be addressed and clarifies issues of concern. It is important to begin letting women in your local area know about the proposed changes, the potential benefits and what the new service will offer them. Consumer support organizations are only too happy to help circulate good news. Women booking for care can also be informed directly using written material that outlines the options available to them and also provides choice. Prior to the launch of the service itself publication via the local media is also beneficial but needs to be handled sensitively.

Staff selection and skill mix

At the early stage of an innovation in the organization of practice different and new skills are required. As these innovations, such as group practices, become the norm recruitment should open up to include midwives with a range of skills. When group practices start, many of the midwives will feel that they are practising under a microscope, with every *faux pas* or mistake observed, but triumphs often passing unnoticed (although rarely are they unnoticed by the clients). In fact, success can bring its own problems; it is sometimes resented.

We believe that midwives need to volunteer to practise in this way and should go through a process of selection to take on the increased professional responsibility, autonomy and accountability that is involved in individualized care and caseload management. In Queen Charlotte's and Hammersmith Maternity Service the action group found it beneficial to advertise posts. Support from the human resources or personnel department from an early stage is important. Also, bringing in representatives from the industrial relations department of the professional organization will help prevent disputes later. Disputes are the last thing needed as the innovation gets off the ground.

To achieve successful selection 'person specifications' define the qualifications, experiences, skills, styles and qualities required of the postholder. For such an innovative post, prior to determining what needs to be included in the specifications we found it helpful to establish a working party that included a member from the personnel department, the clinical leader and elected professional colleagues, as well as a consumer. We found that in-depth discussion with others provided clarification of the type of midwife required for the post itself. Person specifications also focus on qualifications and length of experience. However, we felt it was important to acknowledge the sensitivity, personal attributes and professional skills required of the new type of midwife. Following clarification of these fundamental issues the job descriptions can be drafted outlining the post itself, accountability lines and key tasks to be undertaken within the role.

In order to manage an effective and efficient service, midwife numbers need to be balanced in response to the service needs and the anticipated workload. Birth trend statistics can be used as a guide to achieve this objective including past and future projections. It is important also to address the socio-economic and demographic profile of the catchment area(s) thus defining the needs of the population. Governmental directive initiatives, service specifications, and purchasing targets also require consideration as well as how they can be implemented. When this has been done posts are considered within the organization as a whole and in the light of the available resources.

We believe that group practice design, midwife partnerships and on call systems need to be agreed by the midwives themselves. When deciding upon the shape and number of group practices, the educational and development needs of the midwives and students should be considered, as well as the impact of the new style of practice on other professionals remaining within the existing organization. It emerged that group practices of six suited our criteria, as recommended by several authors (Flint & Poulengeris, 1987; Wraight, *et al.*, 1993). In the Centre for Midwifery Practice the midwives work in partnerships within the group practices, as recommended by Ball, *et al.*, (1992). Co-ordination of group practice activities can be achieved through identified responsibilities, and identified co-ordinator rotational posts enable all midwives to exercise and acquire managerial skills. Another advantage of rotating posts for co-ordinators is that it prevents work overload, especially in the early days for those undertaking the role. These co-ordinators also work in partnership with the clinical leader and provide a supportive network. Having identified midwives as a link for the clinical leader, feedback of information is enhanced, especially relating to the group practices themselves and working methods undertaken within the community.

Staff and new appointments

Advertising of posts should be directed by the personnel department. Timing for recruitment should consider processing, shortlisting and access of information from the clinical project leader or appropriate personnel for the prospective midwives prior to interview.

The appropriate constitution of an interview panel is of paramount importance to the success of the interview and selection process itself and we found it beneficial to include a consumer to represent women's views. At Queen Charlotte's and Hammersmith Maternity Service an exploratory workshop was established by an independent facilitator to enable the midwives to explore attitudes and philosophies, although this was not used as part of the selection process itself. The purpose of this activity was to enable the midwives to focus on their own and group beliefs and the needs of the women who determine their practice. This approach also allowed midwives to de-select themselves if they felt this pattern of working was not for them at this stage, having fully explored what might be expected of them.

During the interview itself, the approach adopted needs to be founded upon the person specification and job descriptions, covering the managerial, educational, research, practical and consumer components of the post. During the interview discussion can include clarification of what is expected of the midwife working within a new style of practice that focuses on women rather than the service. Even though an interview is a formal process it is equally important that candidates are able to relax and express themselves so that the exchange of information should be such that both parties can make a decision about suitability for the post. Undertaking such a fundamental change in practice requires stamina and determination as well as a belief in the philosophies and principles of practice. Working ethos and practices are challenged and midwives need to re-think their management of time and lifestyle. The psychological challenge is perhaps the largest obstacle to overcome. It takes time for midwives to understand that it is acceptable not to report for duty at 8 AM every morning and not be seen on the hospital premises for several days as care is directed into the community. Truly working with women does not fit into a 9–5 pattern. Actually working through the role and personally experiencing the dilemmas involved enables midwives to re-shape their day and working practice. This fundamental change does not occur overnight; it is the hardest aspect of the role for midwives to adopt.

Following selection, individual development needs are identified to provide support for the group practice midwives, thus enabling them to achieve their goal. This can be achieved in consultation with the clinical leader or/and lecturer/practitioner (if in post). Just like the clinical leader, the group practices, once established, also need to identify their own professional, development and supportive systems and networks. Self-selection of midwife partnerships is beneficial and skills, attitudes and experiences can be matched by the midwives themselves. Individual partnerships and group practices need to meet together on a regular basis so that the feeling of isolation is minimized. Practising in such a unique way may mean that midwives will not meet up with their colleagues for several days if time is not allocated for that purpose. Despite regular telephone communication personal contact is very important, especially in the early days.

Now you are there: forming the groups

The formation of the group practices is one of the most important tasks. The group becomes the work unit, with a degree of interdependence between groups. If the group is not functioning and effective, individual practices will suffer. Groups need to share and allocate caseload and workload, share ideals, form their own culture, develop aims and objectives, and support each other.

It needs to be recognized that cohesiveness and group dynamics do not develop overnight and the four stages of group development – forming, storming, norming, performing – should be borne in mind (Tuckman, 1965). Even though group practices are established the midwives should not become dependent upon this structure and should still maintain and foster their own independence. Group decisions can incorporate individual ideas founded upon previous experiences (both life and professional experiences) gained from elsewhere and these can be framed within the overall philosophy of the service. Awareness of potential conflict with the wider organization enables the midwives to adopt strategies for coping should the need arise.

For group discussions to be effective it is beneficial if midwives feel comfortable and free to express their views and feelings so that they can offer constructive criticisms relating to clinical practice. A system of peer review facilitated by the clinical project leader or lecturer practitioner provides a systematic approach to evaluation of practice, promotes reflection and leads to excellence in clinical practice. It is essential to remember that the new style of working is new to all. Therefore, especially in the early days, increased support is essential. Developing a conducive environment and providing explicit support both within the group practices and in the senior midwifery management group enables this to happen. In the early days of team midwifery in Kidlington, it was important for the midwives to meet regularly. This was not only to discuss individual women and cases after on call, but also to reflect on some of the good aspects of the work, for example, a lovely delivery as well as some of the bad experiences including inevitable tiredness after many calls.

At Queen Charlotte's and Hammersmith Maternity Service with the start of one-to-one care the first morning of the new service was spent over breakfast with all the midwives assembled together. There were feelings of apprehension, excitement and desire for the midwives to commence practice. Everyone wanted to know who would be the first to accompany a woman and support her in labour and what it would be like to be with a woman where a relationship had developed between woman and midwife.

On Vicky's first day of team midwifery in Kidlington she was called out to visit a woman at home and subsequently accompanied her into hospital when she was in established labour. Reaction from colleagues (and Vicky!) on the labour ward included surprise at how quickly the new system had been put into action.

Sharing of experiences and feelings during the change of service is a new philosophy. The clinical leader needs to encourage midwives to believe that it is acceptable to express how they feel. Traditional systems have failed to allow professionals to de-brief and the more senior they became the harder it has been.

We suggest that it is important to remember you are human too! Home, friends and social life are just as, if not more, important than work. They should complement one another, and if in proper balance, will enhance behaviour at work and play.

Caseload management

When midwives are allocated to wards and departments, they respond to the workload as it arises. With caseload management, work needs to be planned. The group leader may be the best placed to co-ordinate the caseload allocation, ensuring the workload is evenly distributed, and that the caseload is allocated according to the expected dates of delivery of individual women.

When considering workload distribution within partnerships and group practices various models can be adopted. We found it beneficial to draw upon our own personal and time management experiences, as well as information provided by established models (Ball, *et al.*, 1992). The clinical leader is responsible for ensuring midwives are confident and competent in developing and adopting effective strategies so that all aspects of the role can be incorporated into their day-to-day workload balanced against periods of time for self and student education, reflection, group work and relaxation. It is fundamental that workloads are based around estimated dates of delivery. At first glance this appears a simple rule to follow. However when 60 general practitioners are considered, two hospital sites, geographical areas, midwives' holidays, study leave and social life, the picture changes! The skill of caseload management is complex and mastering that skill is a challenge in itself. Effective time management is essential. A midwife coming out of the traditional service, especially from a junior role, has so much to learn at once. Admiration for midwives who embark on such a change is deserved and their commitment should be recognized.

Regular meetings involving all midwives are beneficial and encourage two way dialogue between the clinical leader, lecturer practitioner, researchers and the midwives themselves. This also leads to smooth running of the organization, review of practice, clarifying of thoughts and provides a mechanism for expression and relief of stress. Midwives carrying caseloads predominantly work within the community with the women they care for, and as such they become increasingly aware of the individual needs of women and their families within that community. Regular discussions between the clinical leader and group practices provides a mechanism by which these needs can be met and by which future service development can be planned to reflect this.

Politics and risk factors

Up until now we have described the practicalities, the nuts and bolts of setting up group practices. But the background to this change, the politics of change which is profound, which alters structure, culture and power relationships, requires separate consideration. The clinical leader is a political activist in this change, literally on the sharp edge. The role cannot be fulfilled without understanding the politics which are an inevitable part of any change, but particularly change like this.

To move to woman-centred care, away from highly technical approaches, to a midwifery emphasis and away from a medical model, requires real political astuteness. Inevitably, it seems, tension arises between the obstetrical and midwifery approaches. The clinical leader needs to view situations from all sides, For the majority of women pregnancy is viewed as a normal physiological and major life event. Professionals can view this differently, based upon their own experiences and the nature of their training. To generalize, midwives perceive pregnancy as a normal life event in a social context, until proved otherwise. At the other end of the scale obstetricians view pregnancy as abnormal until normality is proved retrospectively. General practitioners are found somewhere between the two; whilst acknowledging the woman in her social and familial role they also acknowledge the medical argument, 'normality retrospectively'. As we travelled through our journey of change we found that this variation of beliefs can lead to a lack of understanding of each others professional roles within the maternity services. As well as our own experiences evidence to support this range of beliefs can be found within recent governmental and professional reports (Winterton Report, 1992; RCOG *et al.*, 1992; Cumberlege Report, 1993).

Within the current maternity/obstetrics services, desired maternity outcomes are medically determined by morbidity and mortality rates with reduced emphasis on the sociological, psychological and satisfaction outcomes for the women themselves. All too commonly the interests and cultural needs of women during childbirth are ignored. Throughout our discussions with professional colleagues the common message and theme that filtered through appeared to be that professionals from each group are determined to perceive the change in service from their own individual perspective rather than focusing on the need for change. Throughout the negotiation process it is important to stress that the change in service is for the women themselves and not for one particular professional group.

Politics are about different ways of achieving often similar ends or goals. To highlight this point, Morgan (1986) states that politics arise when people think differently ... and want to act differently. This creates a tension that needs to be resolved through political means.' He suggests varied ways in which this can be done: 'autocratically (we'll do it this way); bureaucratically (we're supposed to do it this way) or democratically (how shall we do it)'. The approach taken inevitably focuses on the power relations between those involved. Conflict is therefore inevitable whenever interests collide. This is in some way comforting because it is an essential part of a dynamic organization. This does not make for easy working at times and can put individuals under great stress, especially if the conflict feels personal, which at times it will.

Risks and safety

Issues of risk and safety are often at the centre of the debate.

Throughout the planning of the service the initial debate with professional colleagues usually centred around:

- Why the need for change?
- The extent of the obstetric risk.
- What the definition of risk should be.

At the Queen Charlotte's and Hammersmith Maternity Service the action group found it helpful throughout these debates to form a working party to concentrate on this issue. This exercise was extremely helpful and promoted discussion on the wider issues of midwifery and social support, enabling a consensus agreement to be reached. It also highlighted the lack of clarity of definition.

From the experience of both of us we believe that organizationally and managerially, it is easier to plan a service which suits all categories of women regardless of potential risk factor, as it ensures that the needs of all women are met. In our experience women who require special support from a midwife usually have had a risk factor identified at booking. If the midwife is responsible for midwifery care planning regardless of risk factors, dialogue and exchange of information between all groups is enhanced as the named midwife is the link professional and woman's advocate. Midwives are not working in isolation and the roles of obstetrical and medical colleagues need to be acknowledged and respected.

Other colleagues are also a knowledge source for midwives. During the planning phase decisions can be taken to the management and advisory group for final clarification and decision making thus providing formal approval.

Power

The whole emphasis of the change, the empowerment of women, is the crux of political difficulties which arise. Embarking upon such a fundamental change in the way midwifery services are delivered, the power base of professional colleagues needs to be considered and at times challenged. 'Power is the ability to put an idea into practice' (Page, 1993). One intention of these changes is to release some of the organizational/professional power and place it with women themselves enabling them to have a voice. Power and responsibility also need to be devolved to the midwives so that they can become true advocates for the women they care for, working together with women in the true sense.

Release of power is difficult and uncomfortable for those who are used to working within the traditional service. The clinical leader and midwifery management team need to convince those involved that the way forward is the right way and most of all that it is what the clients themselves want.

Gender

Within the NHS the issue of gender is an important one, especially in relation to maternity care. There are many common traits traditionally considered to be associated with being male and female in Western society. For example people stereotype the logical rational male and the intuitive emotional female (Morgan, 1986).

We believe that qualities and traits can apply to both sexes, and different traits will emerge in all individuals. In maternity services the gender issue is important because the clients are all women and the term midwife means 'with woman'. Gender bias however is found in language myths and within the culture of organizations which can exclude either sex, just by the nature of the specific working methods of the organization. Feminist critiques of health care have challenged it on this very issue including the male dominance over maternity care (Oakley, 1980). In order to tailor a service to meet the needs of women and their families, it is necessary for the women themselves to be heard. For the service and new style of midwifery practice to be successful the needs of women must be the central focus. Challenging the *status quo* in this area is quite unique.

Working together

Of course we must work collaboratively with medical staff but this does not imply a subordinate position. It is foolish to let them prevent you from reviewing and initiating change in maternity care. We will not be prescriptive. In an attempt to change the way maternity care is provided, midwives get to know medical colleagues in their own areas and learn the appropriate negotiation skills required, as well as the appropriate style that needs to be adopted to suit the audience that they are addressing.

Any honest account of the changing power relationships between women, midwives and doctors must acknowledge theories of power relationships and the conflict which arises out of them. Midwives and doctors are both professionals and employees. This dual role immediately causes conflict. As professionals we are taught to make our own decisions, have our own opinions and be treated as equals, yet, as employees we have a contractual obligation to our employers and have to interact with other professionals whose opinions may differ from our own. At the same time we are equally accountable to the system and the women we serve. Independent midwives 'escaped' from the NHS system in order to practise what they believed should be available to women without the constraints of the system; as such they 'voted with their feet'. In order for a woman-centred service to survive within the NHS, midwives and doctors need to work closely together and respect each other's role within that service. Throughout our discussions during the process of change the following opinions have emerged.

Obstetricians have expressed concerns relating to safety and morbidity and mortality outcomes within the maternity services, alongside debate surrounding options for place of birth. We have experienced differing strengths of opinions. Some obstetricians have acknowledged that the new style of practice is the way forward, others believe midwives are not ready or should not take on increased autonomy and responsibility. Liability arguments have featured prominently on the agenda and lack of clarity about the role and legal status of the midwife has often emerged. In some incidents it has been apparent that power bases are being challenged or threatened and this is applicable to a proportion of members of all professional groups, other midwives included.

Discussions with general practitioners have highlighted their concern about perceived erosion of their role as the central focus of care not only of the women they serve but the family as a whole. Those with midwife attachment have been reluctant to relinquish this arrangement believing that the midwife belongs to the surgery. If a midwife has not been practice-attached the idea of introducing the midwife into the primary health care team has been welcomed. The organization of caseload management for midwives is new to general practitioners. Sometimes they do not understand it, being used to midwives who staff clinics, so they cannot always understand why midwives cannot call on more women than the caseload allocation allows. Envisaging several different midwives accessing premises poses particular problems including communication, relationship and practical issues. All of these potential problems need to be addressed at local level on an individual basis with the clinical leader co-ordinating discussions and solutions.

Despite initial reservations most general practitioners have been happy to provide access to their premises for midwives for antenatal care provision. Transferring antenatal care into the woman's home has evoked differing responses. Maggie found in discussion with general practitioners that they believe that women are safer being cared for by midwives within general practice surgeries or the hospital, rather than in the woman's own home. The underlying rationale behind this view is confused and unclear. But eventually there is an acceptance of the new approach. Many hours are spent talking to general practitioners therefore it is essential that the clinical leader fully researches the range and variety of general practitioner services within the health authority and the particular socio-economic and demographic factors within the catchment area. General practitioners need to trust that the clinical leader and the management team understand what goes on within their community and who works there.

Health visitors on the whole welcome caseload management within the community, viewing the concept of continuity as similar to their own method of working, and the change in service delivery has been viewed as an enhancement on present service provision. When all the professional groups work and communicate well together the benefits to women are enormous, especially for those with difficult emotional and/or social needs.

Unless there is a 'big bang', and the total maternity organization changes overnight during the time of change there will be two services running side-by-side. Balance and acceptance of both services will be achieved if they are acknowledged on their own merits, and effective lines of communication are maintained. Conflict can be managed using the appropriate mechanisms tailored to the individual situation (Crawley, 1992).

The power of persuasion

Challenging people's opinions and values is not easy and is fraught with problems. Encouraging dialogue with all professional groups is an essential ingredient to success. All professional groups need to examine what they do and why they do it. This can be extremely painful and stressful. However, it can reap rewards for all those concerned and a greater understanding of each other's roles and needs. It is an essential part of reviewing the purpose, goals, and effectiveness of our care.

So what makes for good negotiation and how can the process be constructive? Kanter (1984) suggests we need to move away from hierarchical systems and move to a new attitude of openness, innovation and flexibility in order to manage change effectively. As the clinical leader you will often be in the position of being a facilitator and the focus for negotiation. This is because it is a multifaceted post: leader, manager, employee, professional and scapegoat. It is surrounded by people who range from helpful, enthusiastic and committed through to indifferent and belligerent and downright unreasonable and combative. It is also fair to say that individuals can be anywhere on this scale at any time, and your friends and enemies may be those who you least expect!

It is worth always being aware of the players in the negotiations and their views. Get to know the people and try to get beyond the stereotypes and prejudices you may have and learn to control them. The clinical leader is in a pivotal position, and it is important to remember that very few people are actually difficult by nature (honestly!). Sometimes individuals will behave in certain ways because they are expected to or perhaps because they or their professional group feels threatened. This is true especially when there is a conflict of interest and/or an atmosphere of uncertainty. We have found some simple rules really helpful. Be courteous – no matter what is happening. Simple hellos, thank yous, and smiles make all the difference – remember people may be extremely nervous. Try and make the situation as relaxed as possible. When entering negotiations set your ideal (the best you can hope to achieve), your minimum (the least you are prepared to settle for) and your target (what you realistically have a good chance of achieving). The clinical leader should not expect to have immediate success. Negotiation can and does take time, and more than one meeting may be required to achieve results. It is also advantageous to follow up on outcomes.

A key negotiation skill is to listen truly to what the other person has to say. Contentious issues need to be thoroughly thrashed out. This often pays dividends in the long run, helping both sides reach some under-standing, if not agreement. Fully assess what the other person is saying and why. Not everyone has the same level of skill when communicating their thoughts and ideas so if it is not clear what is being said seek further clarification. Wherever possible, it is beneficial to try to take the wider view. Good negotiations are generally achieved with a little give and take. However, it is important to be well informed and capable of providing a good counter-argument if challenged. It is also important to summarize what has occurred during discussions and agreements that have been made.

Bring along appropriate individuals to the negotiation, but tell the others involved so they too can bring along their supporters. It does not make for useful negotiation to have 40 midwives and one consultant around a table! As a general rule you do not have to do all the work. It is not a sign of weakness to ask for help and advice; in fact it is a positive attribute and provides energy and helps gain strength.

Conclusion

We hope we have given you a flavour of our experiences and some of the dimensions of the role of clinical leader. We feel it is important to emphasize once again, the role is open to adaptation dependent upon local, financial and organization constraints and benefits.

For ourselves we believe that working in this way has enhanced our work as midwives and has begun the process of enabling women to be fully aware and involved in their care. We would like to see the growth of similar ways of working leading to a fundamental change nationally, for all women and their families.

We both acknowledge that the post of clinical leader is not for the faint-hearted, but the benefits are numerous professionally in the development of our clinical and managerial work, and personally.

Chapter 12
Being and Becoming the Named Midwife

The named midwife: what does it mean?

'A named qualified nurse, midwife or health visitor responsible for each patient. The Charter Standard is that you should have a named, qualified nurse, midwife or health visitor who will be responsible for your nursing or midwifery care.'   (*The Patient's Charter*, DOH 1991)

The main focus of this book is about finding ways to provide sensitive individual care to women around the time of the birth of their babies. The key to achieving such care lies in finding a way for midwives to get to know the women and families in their care as individuals, and to follow these women through pregnancy, labour and birth, and the early weeks following birth. The aim for the midwife is to develop a relationship with individual women, a relationship of trust. As we are reminded in the Cumberlege Report 'When a woman is having a baby, nothing can replace the support of a known and trusted professional. Many women described the reassurance of seeing a familiar face at critical points, when they were anxious and when complications arose, but especially when they went into labour' (Cumberlege Report, 1993 paragraph 2.3.1).

Over the next five years maternity services in England will be seeking ways to ensure that 'Every woman should know one midwife who ensures continuity of her midwifery care – the named midwife' (Cumberlege Report, 1993, p. 70). The Cumberlege Report reminds us that:

'Wherever possible the named midwife should be located in the community. This neighbourhood midwife should feel comfortable practising both in the community and the hospital. The principle that the midwife should be with the woman when and where she is needed is of crucial importance.'   (Cumberlege Report, 1993, p. 2.3.4).

This will require a change in the organization of care so that many midwives will carry caseloads, but will also require that midwives practise in a fundamentally different way. Being the named midwife for a number of women will require a different organization of work patterns, and a greater personal commitment. In this chapter I talk about ways that midwives might manage this greater commitment, and find it rewarding. I also talk about ways that midwives might organize taking on caseloads within their units.

Being the named midwife

The essence of the new midwifery is to recognize that the relationship between the woman and her midwife is of great importance in itself. The midwife is both friend and professional to the woman she cares for around the time of pregnancy and birth. Relationships are probably the most important part of a human's life. The interaction between two human beings is what brings pleasure, a sense of well-being and of course frustration and spice to our lives. It might be worth making a list of up to ten close and loving relationships that you have: husband, mum, sister, son, daughter, best friend, old school friend, neighbour. What are the characteristics of these relationships? What makes them so meaningful for you?

Firstly, the other person is someone who loves you too, who loves you back in the same way that you love them. The other person is somebody who is familiar and so you know normally how they are going to react to certain situations in life. You can trust them and feel at ease with them.

Friends and family make you feel good about yourself because they love you and because they care about you – they make you feel loveable and cared for and valuable. They are interesting and you like to hear their news and their gossip because they bring you a new view of the world which is different from your own.

All human beings appear to need continuity in their lives. Most of us having found a hairdresser who does our hair in the way that we like, tend to always go to that hairdresser and time our visits so that a particular stylist will be able to do our hair. It is the same with the car. We normally take our car to the same garage and to the same mechanic. We trust the care of our teeth to the same dentist, our health to the same doctor. Humans need stable and continuous people in their lives; for close personal relationships we do not appear to need huge variety.

Is it at all surprising then, that when a woman is at her most vulnerable she should want somebody she knows with her throughout the process? After all she is going through one of the most demanding physical upheavals in her life, when she is changing her role from being a woman unencumbered into being a mother of another human being. This is not something that we feel that we need variety in. We need continuity – we need a relationship.

We only need to look at other mammals who will stop labouring if they are disturbed by an animal they do not know, to be able to see that knowing those present at labour is exceedingly important to other mammals – why not to humans?

Those who are familiar with the labouring habits of the domestic cat or dog, and those who are familiar with other labouring mammals such as cows, pigs, sheep and horses will confirm that the usual time that mammals labour is during the night, that the mammal has to be undisturbed whilst in labour or labour will stop, that the mammal usually labours on its own and if anyone is there it must be someone familiar and unthreatening or the process will stop. Many mammals choose the smallest and most private space possible (for instance, the cat will choose the airing cupboard or inside a wardrobe) and universally the birth takes place in the dark. Ask any midwife where a great many births take place when a woman is in labour at home. She will tell you that it is in the bathroom or lavatory – literally the smallest room. For a generously-proportioned midwife it can be rather a squash!

Women have been asking for continuity of care for many years. They have never asked to be looked after by a team, they have asked for one person, someone they can build a relationship with during their pregnancy, who remains with them during labour and afterwards.

As far as midwives are concerned, for a woman to have just one person may be too demanding on that single person, and they would prefer to provide her with at least two people. Nonetheless, it is one person that women have asked for. In a collection of quotations from women's writings, women's studies, women's magazines, as well as medical reports and journals from 1978 the same refrain is heard throughout. For example, *Parents Magazine* ran a survey to elicit responses about the maternity services. There were 7500 responses to the 1983 survey, which showed that,

> 'Mothers would like antenatal, delivery and postnatal care to be provided, as far as possible, by the same people. Again and again, letters expressed the anxiety that arises when seeing a different doctor at each visit to the antenatal clinic, and at being delivered by total strangers – sometimes two different shifts of total strangers if a woman has a long enough labour.'
>
> (*Parents Magazine* 1983; 92).

In 1986 there were 9000 replies to the survey published within the magazine, showing similar concerns:

> 'Good communications between parents and the medical staff were helped where women saw the same doctor and midwife regularly . . . most mothers saw different people at almost every antenatal visit and were delivered by total strangers. While full of praise for the care they

received, many women wished they could have had more continuity of care through pregnancy and beyond.'

(*Parents Magazine* 1986; 128)

Reports from government and from professional organizations have recommended the need for greater continuity of care for over a decade (Short Report, 1980; RCOG, 1982; ARM, 1986; RCM, 1991; Winterton Report, 1992; Cumberlege Report, 1993). Writers of influence have similarly explored the importance of continuity to individual women (Micklethwaite, *et al.*, 1978; Boyd & Sellars, 1982; Kitzinger, 1981; Melia, *et al.*, 1991). Importantly, the seminal work of Chalmers, *et al.* (1989) which was based on a review of evidence suggested that:

'The midwife is ideally qualified to provide continuity of care, as she is the only health professional whose training relates specifically to both the clinical and the advisory aspects of pregnancy, labour and the puerperium.'

In a list of forms of care which should be abandoned in the light of the available research evidence is 'failing to provide continuity of care during pregnancy and childbirth'. In the new *Guide to Effective Care in Pregnancy and Childbirth* continuity of care for childbearing women is included in the table indicating 'forms of care likely to be beneficial' (Enkin, *et al.*, in press).

Every birth a home birth

When, for medical reasons or because it is the family's choice, the parents decide to give birth in hospital, we should ensure that every family is treated as they would be if they were in their own home (Page, 1988, p. 258). In exploring the idea of the home birth model as one which could change our approach to birth in hospital, we find a different perspective on care, particularly in labour and birth. At home, the woman and her family automatically have power, over their surroundings, over who they admit to the house and to the bedroom, and how they behave. They will eat and drink when they want to, and be able to get comfortable in the way they want. Home is their territory, it is not the territory of the professionals.

The Winterton Report (1992) looked specifically at the environment of the labour ward, with a view to making it more 'homelike':

'The environment in which a woman gives birth is very important. If a home setting is considered as the model on which to base care a hospital delivery unit should:

- Afford privacy.
- Look like a normal room rather than be reminiscent of an operating theatre.
- Enable refreshments to be available for the woman and her partner or companions;
- Ensure the feasibility of the woman being in control of her labour. All case notes should contain the woman's wishes for her labour;
- Enable the woman to take up those positions in which she is most comfortable;
- Enable the woman to have with her a midwife whom she has been able to form a relationship with during her pregnancy'

(Paragraph 328)

The House of Commons Committee considered that home births should be seen as the model on which to base all care and that a hospital delivery room should look like a home and not be reminiscent of an operating theatre. Neither the Winterton, nor the Cumberlege Reports were specifically advocating home births – but that home births should be seen as the model – the basis for maternity care; that a woman and her attendants should feel in hospital that the room she is in, is in actual fact her room; that by taking on the philosophy her attendants will treat her with increased respect, just as they would if they were visitors in her room at home. No-one will enter without knocking and waiting for someone to let them in. No-one will tell her what she can or cannot eat or drink. This will be her decision, as will the position she takes up, which often depends on the comfort of the furniture or the floor surrounding her.

But the homelike approach to birth is more than providing Laura Ashley wallpaper and having people knock on the bedroom door. What has been important about home births in many parts of the industrialized world is that home has been the place where women have been able to gain adequate attention from their midwife, and often this midwife has been someone they know already, that they have a relationship with. In order for women who wish to give birth in hospital to be cared for in this way, midwives will need to organize their practice differently. Midwives will need to take on caseloads rather than staffing wards and departments.

Becoming the named midwife: taking on a caseload

As a profession we need to be looking at how we can allocate our resources and how we can ensure that all women have continuity of care and carer. We need to explore how:

- Women can be enabled to get to know the person who will be looking after them all the way through their pregnancy, labour and the postnatal period;
- Women can be enabled to make choices;
- We can ensure that women are being listened to and that their choices are being respected.

We need to be aware of the factors that enable a woman to feel in control of the whole experience of childbirth. A popular suggestion for providing all the needs expressed by women is that midwives should have their own caseloads.

In the document *Who's Left Holding the Baby* (Ball, *et al.*, 1992), an organizational framework for making the most of the maternity services, written by a think tank at the Nuffield Institute for Health Services Studies, it was estimated that most women would take 45 hours of midwife time throughout their pregnancy, labour and postnatal visits if using the system described by Hall, *et al.*, (1985).

The number of women a midwife can take on as a caseload is between 36 and 40 women a year (Ball, *et al.*, 1992). Flint (1992; 1993) points out that if midwives take on the care of four women per month for nine months of the year they can then enjoy three months holiday and during that time will be able to rest, complete any extra educational needs that they have, and feel invigorated ready for coming back to deal with their caseload.

Rebuilding your confidence

The thought of having 36 women a year to look after feels quite daunting for many midwives. Often they feel that they might not have the necessary experience to be able to care for women throughout every aspect of pregnancy, labour, delivery and the puerperium. This fear is especially relevant when many midwives have been working in one area and feel that they have lost their skill in other areas.

The UK training of midwives is exceedingly thorough and probably one of the most intensive in the world. The midwife has the experience even if she does not feel that she has. But, once qualified, it seems as if our system is designed to make midwives feel unsure of their skills. Perhaps it is because as midwives we always have someone over us. In a hierarchical system the people at the bottom of the heap always feel overlooked and over supervized. Combined with that feeling is the fact that the parameters and the basic values of our maternity services are based on obstetric norms. This means that our whole practice is run on a definition of normality and planned action which is alien to our culture and philosophy as midwives. No finer way could have been devised to increase our feelings of unworthiness and lack of self confidence, but magical things happen once the woman and the midwife become friends. Everything becomes easier, experience grows with the relationship; knowledge is eagerly sought and skills are re-honed – because they are being done for the friend and not for an amorphous mass of unknown women.

One of the other advantages of taking on a caseload within a group practice is that the group can be set up to give each other support in developing skills and confidence. Firstly, different midwives within the group will have different skills and can help each other make up where there are areas for development. Secondly, it really helps to have a colleague/friend you can talk to if you are lacking confidence in a particular skill, or are concerned about a decision you have made.

Being a midwife with a caseload

The provision of named midwives in a maternity service, implies extra accountability and a special relationship between mother and midwife. Organizing the work of midwives through caseload practice is a way of enabling care by a named midwife. The organizing of time and taking on of the caseload is crucial to success and to helping the midwife get enough time for rest and relaxation.

Managing a caseload

When a midwife takes on a caseload of 36 women a year, it does not mean 36 women are on the books at any one time. Figure 12.1 shows a typical schedule. When viewed from December it can be seen that Jane has four women due in December and four women due in January so she will be seeing eight women quite frequently. The November women will have nearly all delivered and she will be carrying out postnatal care on them. She will not be seeing the October women any more and looking ahead she has no women booked for March because she is going to be on holiday. The women due in February she will be seeing

	Jan	Feb	Mar	Apr	May	Jun	Jul	Aug	Sep	Oct	Nov	Dec	
Jane	4	4	*	4	4	4	*	4	4	4	*	4	36
Flo	*	4	4	4	*	4	4	4	*	4	4	4	36
Dora	4	*	4	4	4	*	4	4	4	*	4	4	36
Robyn	4	4	4	*	4	4	4	*	4	4	4	*	36

* = Holiday   4 = 4 Women

Fig. 12.1   A typical annual schedule for a group practice of four midwives.

every two weeks. The women who are due in April and May she will be seeing very four weeks and the women due in July and August are just booking with her. So at any one time she will never have more than about 20 women that she is dealing with. She will be seeing only between eight and 12 women very frequently and these will be the women she has just delivered or who are coming up to delivery. So in this rolling programme she will have the ability to get to know women and to be involved with them but it will be gradual. New women will take over as the old ones slip away and their babies get older.

Working in this way has many joys and benefits. Firstly, because midwives are on call all the time except when on holiday, the way they arrange their work is different from the way work is organized now. They are in charge of their caseloads, and responsible for organizing the way they work. They need to decide which days they will normally try to have without working. For instance, a midwife who wants to have Sunday and Thursday off will not schedule any antenatal appointments for those two days. Postnatal visits on those two days will be avoided when possible, and, of course, the day off would be cancelled if a client goes into labour. Knowing that there is a month's holiday coming up will help here. The theory behind this type of rota is that all off duty is amalgamated into the three months' holiday, but it is still a good idea to schedule in time off during the week while knowing that this does not necessarily happen quite as scheduled.

The midwife may be a morning person and may decide to start antenatal care at 8 AM and try to finish by 4 PM. A late riser will start antenatal or postnatal care at midday, say, working through the evening. A great concert goer, or theatre buff will schedule visits for the day time in order to leave the evenings free. Some midwives seem to prefer to do something every day so that each day is a mixture of time to oneself and time with clients.

As long as there are several treats available during the week the midwife will not find it hard to forgo them if needed at a labour. If only one chance of fun is scheduled for the month it makes it hard to miss. It is also not sensible to decide on a treat at the time of going on it because it can be difficult to think of what to do or where to go unless you have scheduled something in the diary. Friends will not always be free at a moment's notice, but if in your diary you have:

Tuesday – Mary keeping this evening free to go to the cinema with me.
Thursday – Rod keeping the evening free for a sauna with me.
Friday – Joan and Martin to dinner.

You may have to ring Mary and apologize because you have someone in labour and arrange for another date next week, but your diary will be full of exciting possibilities, and buoyed up by a lovely birth you will be

pleased to share a sauna with Rod even if you have been up quite a lot of
Tuesday night.

Dealing with lack of sleep

Some people seem to deal with lack of sleep more easily than others.
Dealing with it would appear to be dependent on one's philosophy of
life in general. If you have been up all night there are two ways of dealing
with it. You can either flop around all day the following day and tell
everyone that you are exhausted and had a horrid day, or you can
pretend to yourself that you have had a full night's sleep and that you are
fine. Working in this kind of way you can cancel your antenatal care for
the morning and go to bed or you can decide to carry on with them if
you do not want to do them tomorrow because you are planning to go
out shopping with your sister for a hat for a wedding.

Many years ago I noticed that when midwives were in love they did
not need sleep. They could stay out most of the night with the beloved
and come on duty the next day looking bright as a button and full of
energy, ready to spend the following night in exactly the same way. The
person who falls into bed exhausted at 10 PM every evening because she
cannot do without eight hours sleep is the same person who can go to
parties night after night without apparent ill effects when she is dating
some luscious guy. Being a midwife may not be in quite the same league
as being in love with Mr or Miss Gorgeous, but a stimulating life can
apparently obviate the need for quite so much sleep. One of the best
ways of helping yourself have enough energy is to have a rest in the
middle of the day. My ambition in life is to have a stunningly active
morning, a rest in the middle of the day, a quiet afternoon and then a
jazzy evening. Having had a rest in the daytime, I will not be too tired if I
am called out during the night.

Being on call

In these days of modern communication systems it is easy to carry either
a portable telephone or a bleeper. Personally I find a bleeper less
intrusive than a telephone. I have a message pager which can be turned
to mute when I am at the theatre or a concert. Instead it flashes at me
when it is going off. Because it holds quite a long message, and I have
trained the women on my caseload to give me a full message, the
message usually goes something like:

'Hello Caroline, Mary here on 071 339 4562. I've been having
contractions every five minutes since 6 PM but they aren't that strong.
I'm planning to go out to my antenatal class now but will keep you
posted.'

'Dear Caroline, can I change my antenatal appointment for Thursday to another day as I've been offered some work on that day – Friday or Wednesday would do. Love Daisy 071 299 0613.'

'Hi Caroline, Libby here, 071 693 5422. Have you seen that there is a programme on Channel 4 tonight at 8.30 PM on home births?'

Having this type of message pager means that messages are screened and you can deal with them as quickly or as slowly as is necessary. Most people are near a telephone most of the time. On the other hand the use of this type of message pager is enhanced when the midwife has a car phone too, especially if her patch is large.

High risk? Low risk?

It helps to know the woman wherever she delivers or whatever her medical condition is. If she is a diabetic woman who needs frequent consultations with an obstetrician and physician she will still need a midwife providing her with support during her pregnancy and clinical care during her labour and delivery and postnatally. If this midwife is somebody she has been able to get to know and build up a friendship with it will be a more supported experience for her and much more enjoyable, whereas at the moment she is probably meeting between 30 and 40 different midwives who are all trying to carry out that role but failing for the woman – because to her they are just a sea of faces.

Equally if a general practitioner wants to keep in touch with a woman during her pregnancy there is no reason why the midwife and the general practitioner cannot share care of the woman. The midwife will be able to provide very flexible care so that she can fit in with the needs of the woman, the general practitioner and the obstetrician and always the woman will have access to a midwife she has come to know and trust.

Learning more

Midwives will find that by having their own caseload they will learn in depth about specific conditions. If a woman they are looking after has, for instance, a low platelet count they will find out all about benign gestational thrombocytopaenia, not because they are specifically interested in benign gestational thrombocytopaenia but because Jane has benign gestational thrombocytopaenia and she is now their friend, or Fiona has benign gestational thrombocytopaenia and they have developed a relationship with her.

Taking on caseloads

Figure 12.1 shows a typical schedule for four midwives (Jane, Flo, Dora and Robyn) working in group practice. Each midwife has an annual caseload of 36 women, booked in batches of four per month. The rota is arranged so that each midwife is on call for three months and then has one month off. The holidays are synchronized so that there are always three midwives on call.

The rota assumes that the women will be seen antenatally at a central point – a surgery or a clinic, that when the women go into labour they will contact the midwife by bleep or telephone and that the midwife will assess the labour in the woman's own home (Klein, *et al.*, 1983) and then will deliver the woman either at home or in hospital. Following the delivery the woman will be looked after daily by her midwife wherever she is (either in hospital or at home).

Although the midwives have their own distinct caseloads, they support each other and give back-up as necessary. It is likely that each client will get to know her named midwife's back-up partner. This would give the midwives greater flexibility and allow them to have a weekend away from the practice occasionally.

In order to take on care in this way it will be necessary for groups of midwives able and willing to take on caseloads to identify themselves and join together.

Starting in the unit

Now let us see how this system could be started easily in your unit. Maternity unit X decides that caseload practice will start on 1 January next year and the midwives will begin to book women for their own caseloads from 1 June this year.

In this unit there are 3000 deliveries per year and 105 whole time equivalent midwives on the staff. It has been decided that 84 of the midwives will be having their own caseloads and 21 of the midwives will be working as core staff in the labour and postnatal ward in order to have three midwives available at any time within the hospital. The 21 midwives will be working exactly the same shifts as they do now. They will have to be highly efficient and able to scrub for sections and run the labour ward efficiently. It is proposed that they have adequate back-up staff such as clerks, domestics and assistants to run in theatre, to fetch and to carry, to clean, and answer the telephone.

The 84 midwives who will be having their own caseloads start looking for three other midwives they would like to start work with. A sample rota is shown to them and they decide which line to work. Jane (who works on the labour ward) has a brother who is to be married in March so she takes the line 1. Robyn (who works in the antenatal clinic) thinks that it will be a bit of a muddle in January when the caseload practice starts. She decides to take line 2 so that she is on holiday in January. Dora (a community midwife) does not much mind and is happy with line 3.

Jane starts her caseload (Fig. 12.2)

Jane has been working in the labour ward for some time now, but during June she will book one woman every week. The women will be 12 weeks pregnant and will be due next January. Perhaps she can do this during the overlap in the afternoon (a system which has disappeared from many off duties but could be re-instated for the build up towards caseload practice).

In July Jane will book a further four women. They will be 12 weeks pregnant then, and due in February. She will see the four women she booked in June for routine antenatal care. Thus in July she will have eight women to see antenatally. This will have to be fitted in with her labour ward work and each unit will have to decide how it will work this out. Jane may be given a half day each week in order to see the women during the afternoon but in July and August she will only have eight women to see during the whole month (two per week).

In September Jane will book a further four women and will see the eight women she has already taken on – a total of 12 for the month. In October she will book a further four women who are due next May and will see a total of 16 women antenatally (including her four new book-ings). In November the women due in June of next year come aboard and Jane sees 20 women (including the new bookings during the month of November). In December she continues to see the twenty women, but the woman who are due in January are seen twice, giving her a total of 24 antenatal consultations that month.

	Jan	Feb	Mar	Apr	May	Jun	Jul	Aug	Sep	Oct	Nov	Dec
Jane	4	4	☼	4	4	4	☼	4	4	4	☼	4
												3 6

Fig. 12.2 Jane's schedule.

Dora starts her caseload (Fig. 12.3)

Dora has been a community midwife for many years. During June she will book one woman every week. The women will be 12 weeks pregnant and will be due next January. Perhaps she can fit this into her present schedule because the women may well be women she would have looked after anyway.

	Jan	Feb	Mar	Apr	May	Jun	Jul	Aug	Sep	Oct	Nov	Dec	
Dora	4	☼	4	4	4	☼	4	4	4	☼	4	4	3 6

Fig. 12.3   Dora's schedule.

In July Dora will not book anyone because the women of 12 weeks of pregnancy are due in February when she will be on holiday. She will see the four women she booked in June for routine antenatal care. In August she will book a further four women and so will see eight women (including the new bookings) during the month.

In September Dora will book a further four women and will see the eight women she has already taken on – a total of 12 for the month. In October she will book a further four women who are due next May and will see a total of 16 women antenatally (including her four new bookings). In November she again has no new bookings (because they would tally with her holiday in June) and again sees 16 women during the month.

In December she continues to see the 20 women, and adds on four new bookings – a total of 24 antenatal consultations during the month.

In January she can just slot into the new system, having got her caseload up and running.

Robyn starts her caseload (Fig. 12.4)

Robyn works on the postnatal ward. She decides to see the women she is taking on during the overlap each afternoon. In her ward the overlap has been introduced in order to accommodate those midwives who are building up their caseload. Robyn sees the women in the postnatal ward. There is a single room which is being kept for this purpose.

Robyn books four women in June, who are due in January. In July she books four more and sees again those booked in June, making a total of eight seen. In August another four women are booked bringing the total to 12.

In September Robyn takes on no new bookings because she will be on holiday in April when the women will be due. She will therefore see only 12 women. In October Robyn books four more women and sees the 12

	Jan	Feb	Mar	Apr	May	Jun	Jul	Aug	Sep	Oct	Nov	Dec	
Robyn	4	4	4	☼	4	4	4	☼	4	4	4	☼	3 6

Fig. 12.4   Robyn's schedule.

already taken on, making a total of 16. In November she sees these 16 women and books four more, bringing the total to 20.

By December Robyn is seeing four women out of the 20 twice and also books four new women, bringing the total to 28.

Like the rest of her group practice, Robyn will be able to slip into caseload practice in January. Also as with the rest of her group practice, sometimes the women will see other health care providers such as their general practitioners or obstetricians. Before a woman goes to see them, Robyn will make sure that the woman has another antenatal appointment scheduled with her so that she does not lose women going off to someone else.

Flo starts her caseload (Fig. 12.5)

It has to be said that Flo is much less enthusiastic than the other members of her group. She has been working in the antenatal clinic for many years. She is not confident about working in the labour ward and she feels that she gives a good service already. None of the arguments about how much the women want this sort of service convince her at all. In June Flo does not book anyone (because the women are due in January when she will be on holiday). In July Flo books four women due in February. They are Tracy, Doreen, Theresa and Amelia. In August Flo books another four women due in March, and she sees Tracey, Doreen, Theresa and Amelia, making a total of eight visits.

In September, Flo books another four women due in April, and sees eight previously booked women, making a total of 12.

Flo is working in the labour ward on the days which used to be for booking clinics to increase her confidence.

In October, Flo does not book anyone. (They would be due in May when her holiday is scheduled.) She sees the 12 women she saw last month including Tracey, Doreen, Theresa and Amelia whom she has now seen four times. Tracey has high blood pressure and protein in her urine and Flo gets her admitted to the ward with a nasty case of pregnancy induced hypertension. Tracey is pleased to see Flo, who visits her every day both to help the ward staff with Tracey's care and to give Tracey moral support. Flo begins to see the attraction of caseload practice – it has really mattered to Tracey that Flo is there.

In November, Flo books four women and sees 12 already booked – making a total of 16. She also takes the baby at Tracey's caesarian at 32

	Jan	Feb	Mar	Apr	May	Jun	Jul	Aug	Sep	Oct	Nov	Dec
Flo	☼	4	4	4	☼	4	4	4	☼	4	4	3 6

Fig. 12.5 Flo's schedule.

weeks and spends the next few weeks supporting Tracey while her baby grows in the Special Care Nursery. In December Flo books four more women and sees the sixteen already booked. Three of these women are seen twice as they are nearing the end of pregnancy. The total is now 23.

Flo is now ready to join in with caseload practice in January.

Imagine your own hospital and community carrying on just as it is at the moment, but with the majority of midwives in the process of taking on caseloads. Each week a caseload midwife books a woman who is due in eight months' time. Over the months this midwife does that woman's antenatal care. Gradually, as the months roll by all women will begin to have their 'own' midwife and the old system will fade away. Thus the new system will be integrated. Given the numbers in the illustration in each unit there should be enough midwives spare to be a skeleton and expert staff on the labour and postnatal wards. These midwives can carry on working shift patterns as now.

The rewards

Once midwives have been able to take on responsibility for 36 women a year their practice will be able to develop and they will be able to experience enormous satisfaction and pleasure from their work. Not only will their professional practice develop but because they are in charge of their caseloads and of how to organize them, they will be able to lead full social lives, fitting in their antenatal and postnatal visits around their own needs as well as those of the women they are caring for. Only labours will interrupt their social lives and as there is only likely to be one of those each week for nine months of the year these should not prove to be too devastating. This way of working will enable the midwifery profession to take on its full role and will give women the service they have been asking for for so many years.

The most difficult part

The most difficult part of having a caseload and getting to know a family, especially the woman, is saying goodbye at the end of the postnatal period. This is a woman that you have drunk endless cups of coffee with; this is the woman you have hugged when she cried on day four and admitted that the whole idea was some terrible mistake and she was not cut out to be a mother; this is the couple you spent a long winter's night with in labour. You know them so well, you love them so dearly.

So – do not say goodbye. I usually say on my last visit, 'My husband and I are always willing to accept invitations to a meal.' These usually only come once the family is on its feet again after the birth and they are forthcoming from those people who want to stay friends. In the light of day the feelings you felt for each other are lovely memories – bringing pleasure to your visits round your district and hugs in the street from old clients. Sometimes it is difficult to get around at all if you meet too many people!

This way of working is what women have been asking us for for so many years. By complying with their requests, we shall take our profession into a new stronger era. Because of the closer relationships we shall develop with the women we shall be empowered as a profession. Because of our increased professionalism the status of the midwifery profession will increase. And I suspect that because of the two-way empowering relationship between us and women, that women will be perceived as stronger and a more dominant force in our culture. But perhaps I had better be quiet about that because the sabotage attempts against it happening are strong enough already! Be strong dear midwife – only you can do it!

Chapter 13
Evaluating Innovations in the Organization of Midwifery Practice

Introduction

This book is about the processes and aims of change within the maternity services. Its central tenet is that both the structure and the culture of the maternity services require fundamental change if we are to achieve what is a substantial redefinition of the goals of maternity care, and alter the experience of maternity and its outcome for women.

Contributors to the book have proposed changes which will provide more flexible, sensitive, appropriate and effective care for women and their families. These changes will in themselves require that midwives change and develop their own practice, and should enhance professional satisfaction for the majority of midwives. Evaluation within the renewed midwifery services should be an integral part of the individual midwife's practice. If undertaken systematically and honestly, this evaluation becomes an integral part of reflection in and on practice.

This chapter is about a different level of evaluation, that of entire systems of care. In particular, it considers issues raised in evaluating fundamental changes in the organization of midwifery practice. We explore reasons why such evaluation is necessary, especially when dealing with organizational change, and go on to describe the aims, design and methods of our own evaluation of one-to-one midwifery care; a new approach to the organization of care implemented within the Centre for Midwifery Practice.

The need for systematic evaluation

Evaluation is part of an approach to care in which we attempt to seek as much honesty and truth at an organizational level as individual practitioners are expected to seek at an individual level. This broad-based organizational evaluation is required because individual practitioners, even those with 30 or 40 years' of practice, do not see sufficient numbers of families to ascertain trends, gauge the size of the effect of a treatment or test, or particular organizations of care. Our individual

174

practice might well help us to develop theories, gain insights, and illuminate principles, but it will not show us the broader picture.

When creating change in a service we need to be clear from the outset how the effectiveness of that change will be evaluated. We need to know from the beginning how to answer such questions as:

- Is the change working?
- If it is not, why not?
- Are the effects of the change those that we intended?

Exposing our most cherished beliefs to systematic evaluation is not easy. Anyone pushing forward an organizational change has to believe strongly, possibly even passionately, in what they do if they are to find the commitment and energy required to sustain such work. There is inevitably a tension between believing in what you are doing and acknowledging that your ideas need testing through formal evaluation. But the fields of obstetrics and gynaecology are littered with examples of new treatments which seemed innocuous, or where the advantages seemed self evident, which later turned out to be harmful, or to have no benefit. The most dramatic story of all, a story which is both simple and dreadful, is that of the blindness caused to so many premature babies through the apparently innocuous treatment of turning up the oxygen to the incubator (Silverman, 1994).

The *Effective Care* books (Chalmers, *et al.*, 1989; Sinclair & Bracken, 1992), have set a gold standard for the maternity services, requiring that we seek to understand the effects of our care using methods which reduce the possibility of apparent effects being due to bias and random error. Enkin *et al.* (in press) suggest that single case reports and case series without formal comparison groups (controls), cannot provide a secure basis for making valid judgements about the effects of care. Such studies are subject to a variety of biases that may either mask real differences between alternative forms of care, or suggest that differences do exist when, in fact, they do not (Chalmers, *et al.*, 1989).

Moreover, fundamental change of the sort indicated here requires great commitment from an organization and the individuals working within it, and alters the use of economic resources. It is thus in the interests of both public and corporate accountability that we should be checking to see whether the change is working, whether it is reaching its stated objectives, and whether resources are being efficiently used.

Service evaluations are, however, somewhat different to research studies evaluating the effects of treatment. Many of the organizational changes referred to in this book have already been shown to be bene-ficial, for example, providing the constant presence and support of a trained care-giver in labour (Hodnett 1993(a)). In addition, many of the proposed changes are to meet needs expressed by the public and women using the maternity services.

Another key feature of a service evaluation is that it can offer feedback on and improve the innovation by identifying dysfunctions in the system of care being evaluated. This means that the evaluation need not stand apart from the innovation in the way that experimental research usually does from practice; evaluation can be integrated with the organizational change.

Evaluating service innovations which already have a mandate requires that the innovation itself lead the evaluation, and not vice versa. The pattern of care described in the next section, for example, was implemented for a large section of a service, and it was not possible to allocate women randomly to this care within the service. In addition, resources were not available to use a larger unit for allocation (e.g., postal districts) and conduct a randomized controlled trial across services.

The evaluation of one-to-one midwifery care

One-to-one midwifery care

One-to-one midwifery practice is a policy initiative which aims to provide each pregnant woman with a named midwife who will be responsible for her care antenatally, intranatally, and postnatally, referring her when necessary for obstetric care. The central aim of one-to-one care is to provide an 'individual service to women and their families, respecting their rights, beliefs and values' (Cooke, *et al.*, 1993). The development arose in response to a groundswell of client dissatisfaction, both nationally and locally, with the consequences of medicalized care, which include fragmented maternity care and its associated morbidity. This dissatisfaction with traditional systems of care accompanies growing evidence that continuity of care is more satisfying to women and has improved many clinical and psycho-social outcomes (Flint & Poulengeris, 1987; Garcia, 1993), as well as evidence that trained support in labour and birth offers psychological, social and physical benefits (Hodnett, 1993a; Wolman, *et al.*, 1993).

One-to-one midwifery care has been offered to childbearing women in two postal districts in West London since November 1993. If the results of the evaluation are satisfactory, it is proposed to extend the scheme to the entire Hammersmith Hospitals Trust.

Evaluating one-to-one midwifery care

The evaluation of an innovation such as one-to-one midwifery care marries attempts to be scientific and rigorous with the chaotic world of the political: the manoeuvring, and the need for dynamic and flexible leadership of organizational change. At the end of the process it is necessary to meet the demands of purchasers, the executive, and other stakeholders. These groups and individuals will want to know whether or not the change is working, and whether or not it is giving a return on the investment. This requires a business orientation.

Effective organizational change is dynamic, and because it is dynamic it can be unpredictable and may seem chaotic to those used to a more orderly existence. Evaluation of a service change is in some sense the opposite of a laboratory experiment where all variables are controlled and monitored. Setting up any change in an organization will have a ripple effect, where the change reaches out and affects a range of things. Creating fundamental change, where the very essence of our daily work is being examined, can make it feel as if a tidal wave is set loose. And although all the participants in the change should be clear where they are going and why they are going there, unexpected things always happen (some of them very good).

The capricious nature of organizational change bears upon the evaluation in two ways. Firstly, you may be designing an evaluation at the early stages of planning, consultation and decisions about change. Consequently, you do not even know if the innovation you have planned is going to happen. The change may not be supported, or, it might progress in directions different to those originally planned.

Secondly, change is a complex process of clarifying primary purposes, setting organizational targets, changing organizational structures and the culture of the organization. Along the way it helps to be aware of and to describe the subtleties and richness of the change, which often reveal considerations that were not anticipated. It is helpful explicitly to build this function into the evaluation design.

Notwithstanding these demands, considerations and uncertainties, it is necessary to uphold scientific principles; to seek valid, reliable and richly descriptive evidence in understanding the change and its effects. Ultimately, we seek to understand whether or not this new approach to care is better for women and babies themselves, and if it is what they want. This requires empathy and sensitivity as well as objectivity in our methods and approaches. So the business orientation needs to be embedded in rigorous scientific approaches; approaches which enable us to understand as well as to quantify, and on the basis of which we can be clear and honest about the extent and limitations of our findings.

We set out to develop an evaluation which would combine objectively measurable outcomes, for example, adherence to standards, costs, extent to which continuity of care was achieved and an in depth analysis of the effects (planned and otherwise) of one-to-one midwifery care. The development of the evaluation has been informed and enriched by the collaboration of a diverse and experienced multi-disciplinary group, set up to steer and monitor the evaluation of one-to-one midwifery care.

The collaboration of this multi-disciplinary group, with experience in different methodologies, has challenged our thinking in an important way. During 18 months of work we have experienced great shifts in our thinking, and developed a deeper understanding of the complexities of the evaluation of organizational change, and of ways that the quantitative and qualitative might be combined. Our first task was to ensure we were clear on our organizational targets, and whether or not they had been achieved.

The organizational targets

One-to-one midwifery care involves partnerships of midwives working within group practices. As a system of care it has the following organizational targets:

- 95% of women to be attended by a midwife they know and have formed a relationship with for labour and delivery.
- Low risk women to be directly cared for by no more than six professionals in the course of their pregnancy.
- Over 75% of women to be cared by their named midwife in labour.
- 75% of total antenatal visits to take place in the community.
- 50% of women to have midwifery-led care throughout.
- 75% of postnatal care to be by named midwife.
- No more than five professionals for midwifery-led care in the postanatal period.
- Peer review to be undertaken by practices themselves every two weeks.

Many of these targets reflect those of the Cumberlege Report (1993, p. 70) although they have taken some of them further forward and some new targets have been added.

In our evaluation we need to find out if our organizational targets have been met. If they have not, something has gone wrong. Original expectations may have been too high. There may be unanticipated resistance to change, inadequate planning. This should not be seen simply as success or failure overall. It may be that given the complexity of the task, outcomes might simply not be as expected. For example, it might be that the desired level of continuity of care cannot be achieved, but that women feel more satisfied because they are offered more choice and control. Or it might be that despite achieving continuity of care targets neither women nor midwives are more satisfied. It is a complex social situation. Outcomes need to be looked at as a whole in order to decide whether the change has been worthwhile. You need clear targets but need to be open minded in interpretation, as well as being rigorous.

This may seem obvious but in practice we often lose sight of the forest for the trees. For instance, in many of the team midwifery schemes set up to improve continuity of care, continuity of care was in fact decreased. There was confusion between the process and the organizational goal. People then started to say team midwifery did not work, when the purpose of the organizational change was not team midwifery per se, but improved continuity of carer.

What is the primary purpose of the change?

Although organizational targets might be seen as good in themselves, there is a primary purpose to reaching these organizational targets. The primary purposes in our case were to:

- Improve satisfaction with maternity care, and facilitate positive responses to the baby and parenting.
- Improve satisfaction with the experience of pregnancy and birth.
- Improve breastfeeding rates.
- Reduce the incidence of operative and medical interventions.
- Reduce rates of depression.
- Support and enhance feelings of well-being, both physical and emotional.

These were the main reasons for introducing change in the organization.

Research design

Description and evaluation

It should be clear by now that designing an evaluation of the effectiveness of the change can be quite complex, and should be thought through carefully. When we started to develop our evaluation we were clear about a few things. We wished to make the evaluation 'hard' and statistical enough, yet we also wanted to capture the richness of the change, and to look at the personal experiences of individual families and professionals. We wanted to understand the detail and know the stories to explain particular findings, as well as to get some quantifiable results.

We also had the words of some cynics ringing in our ears: 'it won't be safe', 'we can't afford it', 'midwives can't/won't do it' and 'it will never work'.

We thought we were clear and had been explicit about what it was we were trying to achieve, but as we went through draft after draft of our protocol we realized that although we had a clear idea in our own minds, which we felt we all shared, we were not making our purpose and targets clear to others.

This process of clarifying purpose and goals is crucial. The process becomes a circular one, informing the process of change. And as soon as we thought we had arrived at a clear statement of our aims, and our design and methods, we would find that we were not able to make the inferences that we had expected from our findings given the design.

Over time we came to separate out more clearly our aims, approaches and methods and to understand the strengths and limitations of our design decisions. We realized that our primary aims were to:

- See whether we had reached our organizational targets and to describe the process of organizational change;
- See how safe and cost effective one-to-one midwifery care was;
- Compare its cost effectiveness with that of the system of care it replaced;
- See how satisfying it was for clients and whether it was associated with improved psycho-social outcomes and/or physical morbidity.

Research aims for the evaluation of one-to-one care

Thus the research aims were to:

(1) Collect data regarding client's satisfaction with care, psycho-social status and well-being, and childbearing experiences.
(2) Assess adherence to clinical standards and medical intervention rates (a surrogate measure of safety and morbidity).
(3) Assess use of economic resources.
(4) Describe the process of organizational change through assessment of adherence to organizational targets, and in depth case study of implementation of one-to-one midwifery care.'

(Wilkins, *et al.*, 1994; p. 2)

Research design

These multi-dimensional aims were to be achieved combining three design approaches:

'(1) A target-based approach, to establish the extent to which specific organizational and clinical standards were met and to assess the use of economic resources;
(2) A comparative approach, which in respect of those targets and resources would compare one-to-one midwifery care with the system of care it replaced;
(3) A descriptive approach, to document clients' experiences of, and

responses to, their care, and to describe the process of organizational change and its meaning to professionals.'

(Wilkins, *et al.*, 1994; p. 2)

The following gives some details of the different dimensions of the
research design.

(1) The target based approach

An important aim of one-to-one midwifery practice is to create cultural
change, that is a change in the accepted values of the organization, and
in personal attitudes and approaches. We are creating an explicitly
woman- and family-centred organization. But structural change is the
basis of the innovation and the trigger to cultural change. This structural
change can be couched in the language of concrete targets, which
should of course, be measurable. So, through a process of discussion,
and based on a review of studies, we determined both organizational
and clinical targets. These targets should be achievable, but not set too
low.

The system should be flexible enough to enable adaptations within
the innovation if the organizational targets are not being met. This is
crucial and bears repetition: if the organizational targets are not being
met, you are simply not testing what you set out to test. If, for example,
we set out to increase continuity by setting up teams, but the teams are
so big that continuity is not increased, we cannot say that continuity has
no influence if clinical outcomes are not changed.

Similarly, if we believe that carrying a caseload will increase midwives'
satisfaction, but then find that the caseload is far too big, and because
they are always rushed and exhausted the midwives dislike carrying a
caseload, we cannot say that it was the approach which was found
wanting.

A target-based approach enables us to measure and monitor the
performance of the service innovation without making unwarranted
generalizations and assertions about causality. This shift, from an
experimental approach based on causal inferences to an evaluation
approach which describes the performance of a system of care against
specified targets, was one of the most important advances made in the
course of our advisory group meetings and offers, we believe, an
appropriate and valid approach for service evaluations of this sort.

(2) The comparative approach

Earlier we discussed the need to evaluate the outcomes associated with a
system of care in a way which reduces the possibility of findings having
been affected by bias and random error. The method *par excellence* of
doing this is through the use of a randomized controlled trial (RCT). Yet,
although we accepted the need for comparison between the new system

of care and the system it replaced, an RCT in this context was impractical and probably not ideal for our purposes. Although we could have randomized clients, midwives, or general practices, in reality this would not have been practical or economical.

Methodologically it would have been preferable to use an RCT. But because we were implementing one-to-one midwifery care over a large part of the maternity service, to randomize women or general practices we would have required two separate services within the same community, and could not have reduced midwife numbers in the delivery suite to bring midwives into the one-to-one practices, an impossible expense.

Nevertheless it should be born in mind that bias is likely to affect the outcome or the interpretation of an evaluation where there has not been randomization to the study group and the control group, and that inferences drawn from such studies tend to be more limited.

Although randomization was neither possible nor desirable, some form of comparison was necessary. We decided to compare the effects of the new system of care through comparison between the study group, a non randomized control group, and two historical control groups, one for the study group, and one for the control group. The concurrent control group was matched on socio-demographic characteristics, thus reducing one important source of bias. The historical controls were intended to make a comparison between people who had received a relatively recently introduced form of care with other people who were cared for in a different way during an earlier era. Historical controls do not enable us to make secure causal inferences, but they do give a picture of the change and variations in outcomes which might be associated with the intervention. The historical controls were also intended as a validity check to see whether any changes which occurred within the study and the control group might be due to factors external to the study.

(3) The descriptive approach

In making fundamental change we are redefining the very essence of the organization. Often everything changes all at once. This is not a slow, staged, incremental change, but requires a review of the social purpose of the organization, its values, its relationships, and its systems (Beckhard, 1992). Successful organizations which have and express a clear sense of purpose work through shared values within the organization, values which are lived in practice (Peters and Waterman 1982). If we are to understand the nature of organizational transformation, and the inculcation of shared commitments, and its relationship to the outcomes we observe, it is essential to gain interpretive understanding from descriptive accounts of the process of organizational change. Through this approach we can attempt to describe in a rich way the values and qualities of a particular organization and follow the stories of players in the change, the professionals concerned.

In addition we need to understand the experiences of clients themselves. We need to know what is important to them, to understand their priorities and needs and the social context within which maternity care is delivered. In seeking out individual experiences we gain deeper understanding and insights which may otherwise be unavailable to us. Not only does this inform and enhance our interpretation of statistical measures, but it also sharpens our analytic understanding and helps us deliver a service appropriate to its stated aims. It helps us understand the meaning of values in practice, and weaves into the harder quantitative data a deeper understanding. As Enkin has said, 'Many of the things which count cannot be counted'.

From a quantitative perspective, qualitative work is often perceived to be subject to bias. At the end of the day we are part of a culture which requires us to justify service provision in clinical, scientific and economic terms. But because the questions, the targets, and the outcomes to be measured in such a way need to be narrowly focused, they are likely to miss important qualities, factors, or outcomes. Thus if quantitative measures and qualitative understanding are combined we may overcome some of the weaknesses of both approaches.

Let us illustrate the point. Recently, a general practitioner practising in a deprived area reported informally at the annual conference of the Association of Community Based Maternity Care in Wales, March 1994. Team midwifery had been set up in her area, and a questionnaire had been given to the study group and the comparison group. Although the results of the questionnaire were the same, what differentiated one set of results from the other was that the team midwifery clients sent pages of written comments of appreciation. What was so striking about this was the fact that these woman came from an extremely deprived area, a place where it was often difficult even to find a pen or pencil in the home, and many of the women were nearly illiterate.

When we compile questionnaires, perhaps to measure psycho-social outcomes, it is important to know what we are looking for. The difficulty is that we are only just beginning to understand what more personal and sensitive care means to women, and the effect it may have. We tend to go out looking for satisfaction, without really understanding what that means, so our carefully constructed questionnaires might miss what is the central point for women themselves.

It was for these reasons we decided for the evaluation of one-to-one midwifery care to combine quantitative and qualitative approaches.

We also sought to feed insights from qualitative research back into our quantitative research instruments such as the questionnaire survey. We shall also explore the meaning of the different types of care for women themselves through observation, exploratory interviews, and analysis of letters.

The evaluation of the effects of organizational change and the description of the process of change are complex, and because of the different strands, they require a multi-method, multi-dimensional approach. It seems from the following that four different studies are proposed. In fact, there is an integrity of approach, and interdependence of the data. These different dimensions will require that different methods of measurement and data collection are used.

Data collection

(1) Study of clients' responses to care and psycho-social outcomes

We were aware that the term 'satisfaction with care' raises more questions than it answers. Satisfaction seems to be an incomplete concept when thinking about women's responses to their care. So, through the questionnaire, we are seeking to explore responses to different aspects of care and care-givers, and are attempting deeper understanding of the different meanings of the relationship between women and their midwives, moving on from the work of Wilkins (1993). In addition, because psycho-social outcomes of pregnancy and birth are so important to the woman herself, her care of her baby, and her family, we are seeking to measure whether or not there might be differences in psycho-social outcomes associated with different forms of care.

Questionnaires

Data regarding views and experiences of care and psycho-social contexts and outcomes will be collected using three self-administered questionnaires (one in late pregnancy [approximately 35 weeks], one at the termination of midwifery care and one at three months postpartum), administered on a longitudinal basis.

Satisfaction with care includes the following measures:

- Likes, dislikes and suggested changes to the system of maternity care.
- The quality of the closest professional relationship (in most cases with the midwife).
- Experiences (where relevant) of other systems of care.
- Satisfaction with specific aspects of care.

The psycho-social measures of the mother cover four main areas:

- Emotional well-being (including feelings about the delivery).
- Perceived relationship with her baby.

- Levels of depression.
- Experience of intranatal pain and postnatal morbidity.

In addition, supplementary social and demographic data will be collected including established measures of social class and measures of social support. The questionnaires consist principally of multiple choice questions and Likert scale (a rating scale for subjective values) evaluations together with a limited number of open questions. Many of the questions are taken or adapted from existing instruments and some have been specifically devised for this evaluation. The questionnaires have been subject to wide peer review from a variety of colleagues in the health authority and experts in the field and have been piloted (by self completion followed up with group and some telephone interviews) with a sample of approximately 90 women who have a range of social and obstetric characteristics.

The data from these questionnaires will be supplemented and illustrated with information from interviews and observation, and selected themes from the findings of the questionnaires will be explored through the interviews.

(2) Study of adherence to audit standards

Rather than redesigning instruments to measure adherence to standards of care we adapted them from two sources. These were both instruments which had been validated and tested in a number of situations. One was a clinical audit sheet, Lilford's 101 measures (Lilford, 1989), which measures clinical reactions to risk situations flagged up through the booking history. The other instrument has been taken from 'Midwifery Monitor' (Hughes & Goldstone, 1993), which measures midwifery care as recorded in the clinical notes against predetermined national standards. We made slight modifications to this.

The combination of these tools provides a measure of the efficacy of the system of referral, and of adherence to midwifery specific standards. We shall also be assessing and comparing intervention rates between the two groups. In theory we expect these to be reduced, given that the women receiving one-to-one care are able to have one-to-one attention in labour from a midwife. The meta analysis of trials of support during labour indicate that a lower operative delivery rate might be expected (Hodnett, 1993a). We also hope that because there is some midwifery-led care midwifery interventions may avoid some innapropriate interventions.

(3) Assessment of the use of economic resources

Any change in any modern day health service needs to provide value for money if it is to survive let alone expand, so measurement of adherence to standards and maternal responses are rarely enough in themselves. These need to be accompanied by evidence that the innovation provides good value for money. This is a particularly important aspect of evaluation where changes in the maternity services in Britain are concerned. Although there is no evidence to support the belief, there seems to be a widespread concern that the provision of continuity of carer and more community-based care will result in higher costs. Furthermore, there is an absence of any meaningful information at the moment. In gathering evidence on the maternity services the House of Commons Health Services Select Committee commented on the lack of information on the costs of different systems of care (Winterton Report, 1992).

On the face of it, determining the costs of different systems seems easy. In fact it is quite complicated. This is partly because costs in many services are nominal, and actual costs have not yet been worked out. Cost and price are not always the same.

In the evaluation of one-to-one midwifery practice it was clear from the beginning that the economic aspects of the evaluation were crucial, both to satisfy local purchasers and providers that the use of resources was equitable, and because we were well aware that the use of economic resources in new systems of maternity care is of vital importance to the national agenda of development proposed in the Cumberlege Report (1993).

For these reasons our economic evaluation is being led by a health care economist. The evaluation has three distinct phases:

(1) The establishment of the cost of the service before the initiation of one-to-one care;
(2) The actual cost of one-to-one care;
(3) The extrapolation of the costs of one-to-one care across the whole service.

(4) Study of organizational process

Compliance with organizational targets

Adherence to organizational targets is not particularly easy to measure in a way which avoids bias. Eventually, for questions on number of care-givers, for example, we decided to count signatures from the patient record – not ideal, but this was the most reliable method available to us.

We thought of having the midwives themselves counting interactions, but this may have led to bias in the recording. Furthermore, the fragmented system of care in the non-randomized concurrent control would mean it was almost impossible to have one midwife attend to one woman's audit of continuity of care.

In addition to the audit of records women will be asked their perceptions of continuity of care through the questionnaire, to validate the findings.

In depth case study

In evaluating organizational change valuable insights may be gained from describing the implementation and the effect of the change on those involved (staff within the organization and users of the service). We shall be seeking the stories of different people within the organization, and will attempt to explore and understand what the changes have meant to different players in the story. We shall also attempt to explore the different values held by different individuals and groups. To do this we have kept documentation of the change. We will be observing, interviewing representatives from all staff groups, and examining the diaries being kept by the midwives.

Determining the size of the study

In addition to avoiding the risk of the findings being created through bias, Enkin and others describe the need to have studies which are large enough to avoid the findings being due to the play of chance or random error (Enkin, *et al.*, in press). Studies 'may seem to detect a difference in outcome that was not brought about by the treatment. This false positive is the alpha error, and the possibility of it happening is defined by the p value. Trials may also have a false negative result and fail to find a genuine difference, a beta error' (Lilford, 1989, p. 462). This is particularly important for the maternity services, where small changes may be of great significance. It is also an important factor in setting up evaluations in small units, or in setting up pilot projects where numbers may simply not be large enough to demonstrate a statistically significant difference.

Where there is concern to examine the effects of care on safety, mortality becomes a difficult measure to use within the developed world because mortality rates are so low. Because of the low mortality rate the study to detect effects on mortality would need to be very large indeed. However, levels of operative intervention rates are generally high, and they may be seen as a measure of safe care for the mother (material morbidity). Other surrogate measures of safe care may be used. Within the evaluation of one-to-one care we have examined adherence to clinical standards. Such measures require much smaller numbers.

Interpretation of results and inferences

It took our small group of researchers some time to come to terms with the limitations of the findings which will arise from the evaluation. Even at a time when there is a growing awareness of the lack of absolutes in knowledge, we wanted to be able to say with conviction that (a) led to (b). Instead, we will be able to compare outcomes in the different groups, but we will not be able to say with certainty which interventions led to which outcomes. Neither will we be able to give a full or exhaustive account of the innovation.

We are also aware that we cannot generalize our findings to all subject groups in other systems of care, for they may differ in ways unknown to us. But our evaluation may, if added to the results of others, get us close to an understanding of the effect of similar changes. Furthermore, if the approach extends within the service, taking in larger numbers of midwives, we may be able to estimate the extent to which the selection of particular midwives biased the findings.

Conclusion

In creating fundamental change, we are re-examining the essence of our work as an institution, the purpose of the institution, and the work of the professionals and others within it. We are attempting to redirect our care to work in the public interest, and to improve what we are doing. The evaluation of the effects of such change is an integral part of the innovation itself, examining the process and effects of the change, and in itself adding to more effective processes and outcomes.

The evaluation we have described is more complex than might be needed or possible for others. It is provided only as an example of an attempt to explore the nature and effectiveness of one innovation, and to raise some questions of design and interpretation which are inevitable in the evaluation of organizational change.

Being clear of our purpose and goals, and of what it is that child-bearing women and their families want from us, and then attempting quite simply to see if we are on target to reach those goals and wants is the essence of what we are all attempting to do. If we are genuinely to work with women, to support their needs and work in their interest, evaluating not only our individual care, but also the effect of the organization and organizational change, is axiomatic.

References

Alexander, J., Levy, V. & Roch, S. (Eds) (1990) *Midwifery Practice. Antenatal Care – a Research Based Approach*. Macmillan, London.

Association of Radical Midwives (1986) *The Vision – Proposals for the Future of the Maternity Services*. ARM, 62 Greetby Hill, Ormskirk, Lancashire L39 2DT.

Auld, M. (1968) Team nursing in a maternity hospital, *Midwife and Health Visitor*, **4**, 242–5.

Ball, J.A. (1992) *Birth Rate: Using Clinical Indicators for Assessing Workload, Staffing and Quality in Delivery Suites and Forecasting Postnatal Bed Needs*. Revised and extended edition of *Birthrate* 1989. Nuffield Institute for Health Services Studies, Leeds University 71–75 Clarendon Road, Leeds LS2 9PL.

Ball, J.A. (1993) Workload measures in midwifery care. In *Further Advances in Midwifery – A Research-Based Approach* (Ed. by J. Alexander, V. Levy & S. Roch) Macmillan Press, London.

Ball, J.A., Flint, C., Garvey, M., Jackson-Baker, A. & Page, L.A. (1992) *Who's left Holding the Baby? An Organisational Framework for Making the Most of Midwifery Services*. The Nuffield Institute for Health Services Studies University of Leeds 71–75 Clarendon Road, Leeds LS2 9PL.

Ball, J.A. & Washbrook, M. (1993) Planning: A Firm Foundation for Midwifery Services. Workload Workshop Manual (Unpublished).

Barber, P. (1989) Developing the person of the professional carer. In *Nursing Practice and Health Care* (Ed. by S. Hinchcliff, S. Norman & J. Schober) Edward Arnold, London.

Barrow, C. & Barrow, P. (1988) *The Business Plan Workbook*. Kogan Page, London.

Beckhard, R. (1992) Changing the Essence. Conference Paper 7, *Managing Fundamental Change*. Office for Public Management, London.

Benner, P. (1984) *From Novice to Expert*. Addison Wesley, London.

Boyd, C. & Sellers, L. (1982) *The British Way of Birth*. Pan Book, London.

Brookfield, S.D. (1987) *Developing Critical Thinkers*. Jossey Bass, San Francisco.

Bryar, R. (1991) Research and Individualised Care in Midwifery. In *Midwives, Research and Childbirth* (Ed. by S. Robinson & A.M. Thomson). Volume II. p. 48–71. Chapman & Hall, London.

Bryman, A. (1988) *Quantity and Quality in Social Research*. Unwin Hyman, London.

Campbell, A.V. (1984) *Moderated Love: A Theology of Professional Care*. SPCK, London.

Campbell, R. & MacFarlane, A. (1987) *Where to Be Born? The Debate and the Evidence*. NPEU, Oxford.

CASP team (1994) *Critical Appraisal Skills for Purchasers*.

Cartwright, A. (1979) *The Dignity of Labour?* Tavistock, London.

Chalmers, I. Enkin, M. & Keirse, M.J.N.C. (1989) *Effective Care in Pregnancy and Childbirth* (2 vols). Oxford University Press, Oxford.

Champion, R. (1992) Professional collaboration: The lecturer practitioner role. In *Developing Professional Education*. (Ed. by H. Bines & D. Watson) Open University Press, Milton Keynes.

Cochrane Collaboration Pregnancy and Childbirth Database (1993) Update Software, Oxford.

Cooke, P. (1994) *The Way Forward: Consultation Document on One to One Midwifery Practice*. The Centre for Midwifery Practice, Queen Charlotte's and Hammersmith Special Health Authority, London.

Cooke, P., Bentley, R., Bridges, A., Douglas, J., Harding, M., Jones, B. & Page, L.A. (1993) *The Way Forward: Proposals and Recommendations from the Centre for Midwifery Practice*. The Centre for Midwifery Practice, Queen Charlotte's and Hammersmith Special Health Authority, London.

Cowell, B. & Wainwright, D. (1981) *Behind the Blue Door: The History of the Royal College of Midwives 1881–1981*. Bailliere Tindall, London.

Crawley, J. (1992) *Constructive Conflict Management: Managers Do Make a Difference*. Nicholas Brealey, London.

Cumberlege Report (1993) *Changing Childbirth*. The Report of the Expert Maternity Group. HMSO, London.

Curran, V. (1986) Taking midwifery off the conveyor belt, *Nursing Times*, **87**, 40–42.

Currell, R.F. (1990) The Organisation of Midwifery Care. In *Antenatal Care: A Research-Based Approach*. (Ed. by J. Alexander, V. Levy & S. Roch), Macmillan Press, London.

Darbyshire, P. (1993) In the hall of mirrors, *Nursing Times*, **89**, 26–9.

Davies, J. & Evans, F. (1991) The Newcastle community midwifery care project. In *Midwives, Research and Childbirth* (Ed. by S. Robinson & A.M. Thomson) Volume II, p. 104–39. Chapman and Hall, London.

Department of Health (1989) *Working for Patients*. HMSO, London.

Department of Health (1991) *The Patient's Charter*, HMSO, London.

Department of Health (1992) *Maternity Care in the New National Health Service – A Joint Approach*. HMSO, London.

Department of Health (1994a) *The Patient's Charter: Maternity Services, England*. HMSO, London.

Department of Health (1994b) *Report on Confidential Enquiries into Maternal Deaths in the United Kingdom 1988–1990*. HMSO, London.

Dewey, J. (1933) *How We Think*. D.C. Heath, Boston.

Downie, R.S. (1990) Professions and professionalism. *Journal of Philosophy of Education,* **24**, 47–50.

Drew, N.C., Salmon, P. & Webb, L. (1989) Mothers', midwives' and obstetricians' views on the features of obstetric care which influence satisfaction with childbirth. *British Journal of Obstetrics and Gynaecology,* **96**, 1084–1088.

Enkin, M., Chalmers, I. & Keirse, M. (1989) *A Guide to Effective Care in Pregnancy and Childbirth.* Oxford University Press, Oxford.

Enkin, M., Keirse, M.J.N.C., Renfrew, M. & Neilson, J. *A Guide to Effective Care in Pregnancy and Childbirth.* Oxford University Press, Oxford (in press).

Enkin, M., Keirse, M.J.N.C., Renfrew, M., & Neilson, J. (Eds) (1993) Pregnancy and childbirth module. *Cochrane Collaboration Pregnancy & Childbirth Database.* Update Software, Oxford.

Fardell, J. (1991) Maintaining a high profile. *Nursing Times,* **87**, 50–51.

Flint, C. (1991) Continuity of care provided by a team of midwives – the Know Your Midwife scheme. In *Midwives, Research and Childbirth* (Ed. by S. Robinson & A.M. Thomson) Volume II, 72–104. Chapman and Hall, London.

Flint, C. (1992) Name, Set and Match. *Health Service Journal,* 23 July, p. 26.

Flint, C. (1993) *Midwifery Teams and Caseloads.* Butterworth Heinemann, London.

Flint, C. & Poulengeris, P. (1987) *The Know Your Midwife Report,* Pub 49. Peckarmans Wood, London SE26 6RZ.

Frohlich, J. & Edwards, S. (1989) Team midwifery for everyone. Building on the Know Your Midwife Scheme. *Midwives Chronicle,* March, 66–70.

Garcia, J. (1989) *Getting Consumers' Views of Maternity Care: Examples of How the OPCS Survey Manual Can Help.* Department of Health, London.

Garcia, J. (1993) *Research on Continuity of Carer.* Paper for Consensus Conference, King's Fund and Department of Health, London.

Gary, A. & Pearsall, M. (Eds) (1989) *Women, Knowledge and Reality.* Unwin Hyman, Boston.

Green, J.M., Coupland, B.A. & Kitzinger, J. (1990) Expectations, experiences, and psychological outcomes of childbirth: a prospective study of 825 women, *Birth,* **17**, 15–24.

Green, J., Coupland, B.A. & Kitzinger, J. (1988) *Great Expectations: A Prospective Study of Women's Expectations and Experiences of Childbirth.* Child Care and Development Group, Cambridge.

Hall, M., Macintyre, S. & Porter, M. (1985) *Antenatal Care Assessed.* Aberdeen University Press, Aberdeen.

Handy, C.B. (1985) *Understanding Organizations.* Third Edition. Penguin Books, London.

Heron, J. (1974) *The Concept of a Peer Learning Community.* Human Potential Research Project. University of Surrey, Surrey.

Hodnett, E. (1993a) Support from caregivers during childbirth. In *Cochrane Collaboration Pregnancy and Childbirth Database* (Ed. by M.W. Enkin, M.J.N.C. Keirse, M.J. Renfrew, & J.P. Neilson) Cochrane Database of Systematic Reviews: Review No. 03871, 12 May 1993. Update Software, Oxford.

Hodnett, E. (1933b) Social support during high-risk pregnancy: does it help? *Birth*, **20**, 218–9.

Hodnett, E. (1993c) Continuity of caregivers during pregnancy and childbirth. In *Cochrane Collaboration Pregnancy and Childbirth Database* (Ed. by M. Enkin, M.J.N.C. Keirse, M. Renfrew & J.P. Neilson) Cochrane Database of Systematic Reviews. Update Software, Oxford.

Hughes, D.J.F. & Goldstone, L.A. (1989) Frameworks for midwifery care in Great Britain: an exploration of quality assurance. *Midwifery*, **5**, 163–171.

Hughes, D.J.F. & Goldstone, L.A. (1993) *Midwifery Monitor, Pregnancy Care! Labour Care? Care After the Birth?* Gale Centre Publications, Loughton, Essex.

James, C. & Clarke, B. (1993) Beyond reflection to collaborative practice. Paper presented to the Fourth International Participative Conference, Nurse Education Tomorrow, University of Derby, September 1993.

Jarvis, P. (Ed) (1987) *Twentieth Century Thinkers in Adult Education*, Croom Helm, London.

Jenks, J. *et al.* (1987) *Learning in the Workplace* (Ed. by V.J. Marsick) Croom Helm, Beckenham.

Kanter, R.M. (1984) *The Change Masters: Corporate Entrepreneurs at Work*. George Allen & Unwin, London.

Kilty, J. & Bond, M. (1992) *Practical Ways of Dealing with Stress*. HPRG Publications, Guildford.

Kirkham, M. (1989) Midwives and information giving during labour. In *Midwives, Research and Childbirth* (Ed. by S. Robinson & A.M. Thomson) Volume I. Chapman and Hall, London.

Kitzinger, S. (1981) *Change in Antenatal Care*. A report of a working party set up for the National Childbirth Trust. NCT: London.

Kitzinger, S. (1992) *Ourselves as Mothers: The Universal Experience of Motherhood*, Doubleday, London.

Klauss, M. (1986) Effects of social support during parturition on material and infant morbidity. *British Medical Journal*, **293**, 585–7.

Klein, M., Lloyd, I. & Redman, C. (1983) A comparison for low risk pregnant women booked for delivery in two systems of care: shared care (consultant) and integrated general practice unit. *British Journal of Nursing Management*, **1**, 31–7.

Klein, M., Lloyd, I., Redman, C., Bull, M. & Turnbull, A.C., (1983) A comparison of low-risk women booked for delivery in two systems of care; shared-care (consultant) and integrated general practice unit. I. Obstetrical procedures and neonatal outcome. II. Labour and delivery management and neonatal outcome. *British Journal of Obstetrics and Gynaecology*, **90**, 118–22 and 123–8.

Knowles, M. (1984) *The Adult Learner: a Neglected Species*, Gulf Publishers, Houston.

Lewin, K. (1951) *Field Theory in Social Science*, Harper & Row, New York.
Lilford, R. (1989) Evaluating new treatments and diagnostic technologies in obstetrics. *International Journal of Technology Assessment in Health Care*, **5**, 459–73.

McKinley, J.B. (1972) The sick role – illness and pregnancy. *Social Science and Medicine*, **6**, 561–72.
McPeck, J.E. (1981) *Critical Thinking and Education*. Martin Robertson, Oxford.
Mason, V. (1989) *Women's Experience of Maternity Care – A Survey Manual*. HMSO, London.
Maternity Services Advisory Committee (1982) *Maternity Care in Action*. HMSO, London.
Meerabeau, L. (1992) Tacit nursing knowledge: an untapped resource or a methodological headache? *Journal of Advanced Nursing*, **17**, 108–12.
Melia, R.J., Morgan, M., Wolfe, C.D.A. & Swan, A.V. (1991) Consumers' views of the maternity services: implications for change and quality assurance. *Journal of Public Health Medicine*, **13**, 120–6.
Mezirow, J. (1989) Transformation theory and social action: a response to Collard and Law. *Adult Education Quarterly*, **39**, 169–75.
Mickelthwaite, P., Beard, R. & Shaw, K. (1978) Expectations of a pregnant woman in relation to her treatment, *British Medical Journal*, **2**, 188–91.
Ministry of Health (1959) Report of the Maternity Services Committee (Cranbrook Report), HMSO, London.
Morgan, G. (1986) *Images of Organisations*. Sage Publications, London.
MORI (1993) *A survey of women's views of the maternity services*. Maternity services research study conducted for the Department of Health.
Morris, N. (1960) Human relations in obstetric practice. *Lancet*, **1**, 913–15.
Morris-Thompson, P. (1993) A historical perspective on maternity services and the Leicester Royal Infirmary Approach to the Winterton Report's recommendations. *Journal of Nursing Management*, **1**, 31–7.
Murphy Black, T. (1992) Systems of midwifery came in use in Scotland. *Midwifery*, **8**, 113–24.

National Health Service Management Executive (1993) *Midwife and GP-led Maternity Units*. NHS Management Executive, Department of Health, London.

Oakley, A. (1979) *Becoming a Mother*. Martin Robertson, Oxford.
Oakley, A. (1980) *Women Confined: Towards a Sociology of Childbirth*. Martin Robertson, Oxford.
Oakley, A. (1984) The Captured Womb: A History of the Medical Care of Pregnant Women. Basil Blackwell, Oxford.
Oakley, A. (1991) Using medical care: the views and experiences of high-risk mothers, *Health Services Research*, **26**, 651–69.
Oakley, A. (1992) *Social Support and Motherhood*. Basil Blackwell, Oxford.

Oakley, A. & Hickey, A. (unpublished) Continuity of care and social support. Social Science Research Unit, London. (Quoted with permission).

O'Brien, M. & Smith, C. (1981) Women's views and experiences of antenatal care. *The Practitioner*, **225**, 123–5.

Ong, B.N. (1983) *Our Motherhood*. Family Service Units, 207 Old Marylebone Road, London NW1 5QP.

Oxman, A.D., Sackett, D.L. & Guyatt, G.H. for the evidence based working group (1993). User's guide to the medical literature 1. How to get started, *JAMA*, **270**, 2093–5.

Page, L.A. (1988) The Midwife in Modern Health Care. In *The Midwife Challenge* (Ed. by S. Kitzinger). Pandora, London.

Page, L.A. (1992) Evidence to House of Commons Select Committee. *House of Commons 1992. Second Report on the Maternity Services. Volume II: Minutes of Evidence*, p. 405. HMSO, London.

Page, L.A. (1993) How and who should be monitored: the midwife's view. In *Intra partum Fetal Surveillance* (Ed. by J.A.D. Spencer & R.H.T. Ward). RCOG Press, London.

Page, L.A. (1993) *Midwives hear the heartbeat of the future*. Keynote address, Proceedings 23rd Triennial Congress of the International Confederation of Midwives, Vancouver Canada.

Page, L.A. & Healey, E. (1990) Midwifery by degree: changes in education and service at Oxford. *Midwife, Health Visitor and Community Nurse*, **26**, 364–70.

Parents Magazine (1983). Birth in Britain. A parents special report. A Survey of 7,500 women's views. **92**.

Parents Magazine (1986) Birth: 9000 mothers speak out. Birth Survey 1986 – results. **28**.

Peel Report (1970) *Domiciliary Midwifery and Maternity Bed Needs. Report of the Sub-Committee, Central Health Services Council Standing Maternity and Midwifery Advisory Committee*. HMSO, London.

Peters, T.J. and Waterman, R.H. Jr (1982) *In Search of Excellence: Lessons from America's Best-Run Companies*. Warner Books, New York.

RCOG (1982) *Report of the RCOG working party on antenatal and intra-partum care*, Royal College of Obstetricians and Gynaecologists, London.

RCOG (1982) *Working Party on Antenatal and Intrapartum Care*, Royal College of Obstetricians and Gynaecologists, London.

RCM (1991) Evidence to the Review Body, Royal College of Midwives, London.

RCM (1991) *Towards a Healthy Nation. Every day a birthday*. Royal College of Midwives, London.

RCOG & RCGP (1992) *Working party on training*. Royal College of Obstetricians and Gynaecologists, London.

RCOG, RCM & RCGP (1992) *Maternity Care in the New NHS – a Joint Approach*. Royal College of Obstetricians and Gynaecologists, London.

Reid, M. & Garcia, J. (1989) Women's views of care during pregnancy and childbirth. In *Effective Care in Pregnancy and Childbirth*. (Ed. by Chalmers, M. Enkin & M.J.N.C. Keirse). Oxford University Press, Oxford.

Reid, M., Gutteridge, S. & McIlwaine, G.M. (1983) *A comparison of the delivery of care between a hospital and a peripheral clinic.* Report submitted to the Scottish Home and Health Department. Social Paediatric and Obstetric Research Unit, University of Glasgow.

Robinson, S. (1989) The role of the midwife: opportunities and constraints. In *Effective Care in Pregnancy and Childbirth* (Ed. by I. Chalmers, M. Enkin & M.J.N.C. Kierse). Oxford University Press, Oxford.

Robinson, S., Golden, J. & Bradley, S. (1983) *A Study of the Role and Responsibility of the Midwife.* Nursing Education Research Unit, London.

Rudat, K., Roberts, C. & Chowdhury, R. (1993) *Maternity Services: A Comparative Survey of Afro-Carribean, Asian and White Women, Commissioned by the Expert Maternity Group.* MORI Health Research Unit, London.

Scholes, K. & Kleman, M. (1977) *An introduction to Business Planning.* McMillan, London.

Schön, D.A. (1991) *Educating the Reflective Practitioner,* Jossey Bass, San Francisco.

Short Report (1980) *Perinatal and Neonatal Mortality.* Second Report from the Parliamentary Social Services Committee 1979–80. HMSO, London.

Silverman, W.A. (1994) *The line between living and dying: Medicines dilemma at the end of the twentieth century.* Windermere lecture, 1994 annual meeting of British Paediatric Association, Warwich.

Simkin, P. (1991) Just Another Day in a Woman's Life? Women's Long Term Perceptions of Their First Birth Experience. Part 1. *Birth,* **18**, 203–10.

Sinclair, J.C. & Bracken, M.B. (Ed.) (1992) *Effective Care of the Newborn Infant.* Oxford University Press, Oxford.

Stanley, L. (Ed.) (1990) *Feminist Praxis.* Routledge, London.

Stock, J. & Wraight, A. (1993) *Industrial Relations and Professional Issues in Team Midwifery.* IMS report, Brighton.

Street, A. (1992) *Cultural Practices in Nursing.* Deakin, London.

Tew, M. (1990) *Safer Childbirth? A Critical History of Maternity Care.* Chapman and Hall, London.

The Patient's Charter Group (1991) *The Named Midwife. Your Questions Answered.* National Health Service.

Tuckman, B. (1965) Development sequences in small groups, *Psychological Bulletin,* **63**.

UKCC (1990) *The Executive Summary of the Report of the Post-Registration Education and Practice Project.* UKCC, London.

Van Manen, M. (1991) *The Tact of Teaching: The Meaning of Pedagogical Thoughtfulness.* State University of New York Press, New York.

Vroom, V.A. (1964) *Work and Motivation.* John Wiley and Sons, New York.

Watson, P. (1990) *Report on the Kidlington Team Midwifery Scheme.* Oxford Institute of Nursing, Radcliffe Infirmary, Oxford.

Webber, M. (1947) *The Theory of Social and Economic Organisation.* Free Press.

West, A. (1988) *A Business Plan*. Pitman Publishing, London.

Wilkins, R. (1993) Sociological aspects of the mother/community midwife relationship. Unpublished PhD thesis, University of Surrey.

Wilkins, R., Page, L.A., Stevens, T., Lilford, R. & Pearcy, J. (1994) *Protocol for the evaluation of one to one midwifery care*. The Centre for Midwifery Practice, Queen Charlotte's and Hammersmith Special Health Authority, London.

Winterton Report (1992) *Second Report on the Maternity Services by the Health Services Select Committee*. HMSO, London.

Wolman, W.L., Chalmers, B. Hofmeyr, J. & Nikodem, V.L. (1993) Postpartum depression and companionship in the clinical birth environment: A randomized controlled study, *American Journal of Obstetrics and Gynaecology*, **168**, 1388–93.

Wraight, A., Ball, J., Seccombe, I. & Stock, J. (1993) *Mapping Team Midwifery: A Report to the Department of Health*. IMS Report Series 242. Institute of Manpower Studies, Brighton.

Zander, L. (1982) The challenge of antenatal care: a perspective from general practice. In *Effectiveness and Satisfaction in Antenatal Care* (Ed. by M. Enkin & I. Chalmers). William Heinemann Medical Books Ltd, Spastics International Medical Publications, London.

Index